BECOMING UNBREAKABLE

HOW TO
BUILD A BODY
YOU LOVE TO
LIVE IN

KATE GALLIETT

ISBN 979-8-9851005-0-1 (paperback edition)
ISBN 979-8-9851005-1-8 (e-book edition)

First paperback edition: Jan 1, 2022

Edited by: Laura Gale, of Laura Gale Creative
Cover art by: Rejenne Pavon, of selfpublishingkit.com
Layout by: Ronald Cruz, of selfpublishingkit.com

Table of envelope of function in The Knee as a Biologic Transmission With an Envelope of Function in the Journal of Clinical Orthopaedics and Related Research reprinted with permission.

Published by Fit For Real Life Press in Salt Lake City, Utah, USA

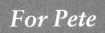

For Pete

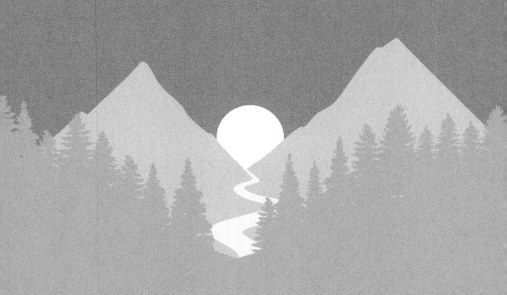

Author's Note

This book comes with bonus material that I've put on a special page on my website for you. This "book bonus" page, which you'll see referenced frequently as you get to part four of the book, has several videos to demonstrate the exercises I'll be teaching you. It also has further information that supports what you're learning as you read, and includes details about how to find out more about the people and things mentioned in this book. You can find the book bonus page at:

www.theunbreakablebody.com/book-bonus

Contents

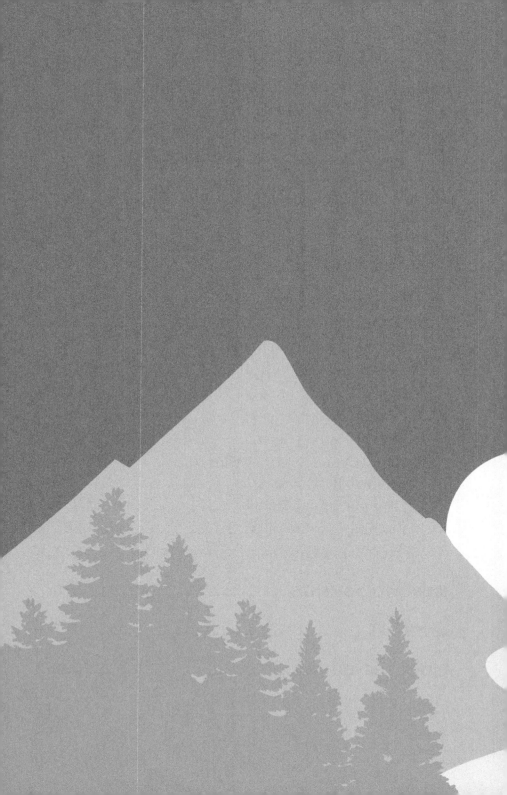

PART ONE:
Your Invitation To Become Unbreakable

CHAPTER 1

'Too Late'

My blood froze. My skin lifted off my body. My muscles started shaking uncontrollably. I heard my voice tell the 911 operator, "We have an emergency, my dad had a stroke, please hurry." I watched out the front room windows, heart racing, desperate to see the flashing lights of an ambulance.

When they finally arrived, I stayed downstairs while they navigated our narrow hallways to gather up my father. As they wheeled him toward the back door, I heard someone yelling. "Kate! Where is Kate? He's calling for you." I went into the back room, looking at him wrapped up in blankets on the stretcher. I couldn't understand what he was saying, but I was there with him until they loaded him up into the ambulance and drove away.

I went to school the next day, trying to hold it together. In the early afternoon, there was a knock on our classroom door and we all turned to see the school receptionist. "I need to see Kate", she said. "Bring your books." She tried to make chit-chat while we made the short walk to the Dean's office. I couldn't make sense of it. 'Why am I going to the office? I know I didn't do anything that would get me in trouble… What the hell is happening?'

Finally, we got to the office and she opened the door. Standing in the office was my mother. "Kate, we have to go, it's Dad." Confused, frightened, out of my body, I said, "Oh, um, okay. I need to get my books out of my locker." She shook her head. "We don't have time."

We ran out to the car and my mother sped like a mad woman all the way to the hospital. We raced in the doors, up the quiet white corridor, only to be caught by three nurses as we neared his room.

"It's too late."

He was gone.

* * *

I had the unfortunate experience of living through my father's death before I was eighteen. While I couldn't make much sense of it back then, it irrevocably shaped my understanding of what 'too late' really means. 'Too late' permeates the conversation about how bodies should feel and what they should be able to do as they age, but the notion that you can reach a point where it's 'too late' to do something for your body is just a pervasive myth. 'Too late' means an action or event is useless or ineffective because it occurs after the time when something could or should have been done.

'Too late' means there's no going back, no re-do, no changing your mind. There are so many options available to you, provided it's not 'too late', and there's actually only one 'too late' moment in this lifetime. Truly, only one, and that's death.

Despite this, a whole lot of people feel like it's too late for them. Maybe you're one of them, concerned that it may be...

- Too late for you to ever recover from joint pain and muscle strains
- Too late to take up a sport
- Too late to go on adventures with your kids
- Too late to change how your body feels

The 'too late' myth even sneaks into everyday conversation in the most subtle of ways, such as, "Well you are 40 now, how did you expect your knees to feel?" The implication is that you're 40 now, and that's too old to have knees that feel good. This myth also shows up when the conversation turns to injuries and aches a person has experienced. "I've got a bum shoulder from an old injury", as if it's too late for you to restore full use of that shoulder.

While it might be true that your knees hurt today, or that you sustained a shoulder injury in the past, what is *more* true is that other than death, there is no situation where it is too late to change anything about yourself. Even if you have a life-altering catastrophic injury, if you are still alive, it is not too late to take ownership of what comes next.

Working with hundreds of clients over the years as a fitness trainer also showed me that there's another myth that creeps in along with the 'too late' myth, and that's the 'too complicated' myth. I've met so many people who would love to feel better in their body, who would love to keep doing the activities they love, and who really don't want to become frail, but they've picked up the myth that bodies are complicated and thus taking care of them is 'too complicated' for the average person to figure out.

There are tissues and joints and systems doing all manner of things in your body every day, and you might not know much about any of them. Health guidance and exercise methods are constantly shifting as new research is done and as old research is revisited, so how can the average person keep up? It's understandable that it feels like a struggle to stay in the know.

The word 'complicated' means that something is not easy to understand because of its intricacy. And your body *is* intricate, but that doesn't mean it's too complicated for you. My friend and colleague, Dr. Seth Oberst, put it perfectly when he said, "When it comes to taking care of your body, it's valuable to know that even though a body is complex, the care of it doesn't need to be complicated."

Both of these myths, that it's 'too late' and 'too complicated', take you out of the driver's seat of your life. They take your personal autonomy — your freedom to know what is right for you better than anyone else and to make choices for yourself, your body, and your life accordingly — and stomp on it. They make other people's voices, ideas, and opinions seem more important and authoritative than your own. They make it more difficult to tune in to the conversation you and your body are having every day. They make it hard to feel motivated to keep trying to make change and improvement for yourself. And they most certainly make it difficult to feel carefree in your body or your life.

And if you've come across these myths and worried they were true, it is completely understandable that you'd feel a sense of hopelessness, frustration, or disappointment. I know, because I had exactly the same experience.

I woke up one day and realized I felt broken in my body. I was acutely aware that the list of things that hurt was growing steadily while the list of activities I was partaking in was shrinking in equal measure. And the real kicker was that I felt this way despite doing everything that's supposed to build a fit body that feels strong and good. I had muscular strength, plenty of flexibility, I could run a marathon and do hard workouts in the gym. But it felt like my body had betrayed me. I felt exhausted and worn out. Something always hurt, and I was constantly sick with infections which doctors told me was "just how I was."

I could distinctly see that I wasn't expanding out into my world and really living life to the fullest. I was shrinking away from it because of how I felt living in my body. The way I was going about fitness and body care was not helping me feel how I wanted to feel, do what I wanted to do, or be who I wanted to be. I wanted to feel resilient, and ready for anything. I wanted to be able to participate fully in every experience that came my way or that I could dream up. I wanted to be fully Me, confidently living in the body, mind, and spirit I had been given. In a word, I wanted to feel *Unbreakable*.

The thought crossed my mind: "But what if it's too late?" It was immediately drowned out as I remembered that I already knew what a real 'too late' moment was, and it wasn't this. And so I went on a journey to become Unbreakable. What I learned along the way became the foundation of all that I teach today to others who want to become Unbreakable, too.

I was able to prove these myths wrong, heal my body aches and injuries, and get rid of the limitations so I could feel how I wanted to feel and do what I wanted to do. I became Unbreakable, and in the years that have passed since then, I've helped a plethora of people to become Unbreakable, too. If we can all do it, so can you.

* * *

7

They say that people are put on your path for a reason, and that was true for me when I met some of the first personal training clients I would work with, several of whom retained me as their trainer for the next decade. These folks were in their 50s and 60s, and they were motivated by activity and adventure.

Ruth was someone who was getting into travel adventures — she was interested in hiking mountains, adventuring in wild places where there was lots of nature to see, and experiencing as much of the world as she could. She was motivated to take care of her body simply for health's sake, but she also was motivated to build her body to stand up to these adventures she was interested in pursuing. She valued being independent and strong, and she never wanted her body to say 'no' to anything her mind dreamed up. She also had grandkids and she was determined to be as active as possible with them when they'd come to visit.

Prior to our meeting, she'd completed some running races, so she wasn't a novice at fitness-based activities, but building strength and fitness for these bigger adventures was a newer goal for her. And at 60, she was hearing the message that it's 'too late' everywhere. People were frequently telling her she should be slowing down now that she was getting older and that she was too old to be so adventurous. But Ruth had no intention of slowing down, in fact she was going to speed up and immerse herself in even more of life as she got older. So she brought me on board for her journey.

And in what can only be chalked up to a perfect, stars-aligning moment, here I was searching for other people who were as hell bent on being Unbreakable and rejecting the 'too late' myth as I was. I hadn't met anyone with the same determination until I met Ruth. Despite our age difference, being able to coach a person to whom I had similar objectives enhanced the work I was already doing to rework how I was caring for my body.

My journey to becoming Unbreakable was enhanced and accelerated because I got to be a part of Ruth's journey, coaching and supporting her as she became Unbreakable and did all the things she loved to do — participating in endurance running races, going on hikes, and adventuring all over the world. Even better than that, she got to be incredibly active with her kids and grandkids at a time when many others her age were slowing down.

Shortly after meeting Ruth, I met Steve. He had always been active, and his pursuits had a wild-child flare to them. He had been a dirtbag (as he lovingly called himself) before being a dirtbag was cool. His forties and fifties were a continuation of the passion he'd always had for adventure, and in those years he summited big mountains, was into rock and ice climbing, played ice hockey, and went on all manner of extended backpacking trips. And he intended to keep that up even as he got older.

Steve was too big a personality for anyone to tell him to his face that it was 'too late' for him, but his own body was speaking up about how he needed to adjust his body care if he wanted to keep doing these things he loved. By the time we met, his training for these adventures required a lot of 'working around' the aches and pains that he was developing, which limited how much fitness he could actually build. He was acutely aware that aches and pains popping up on a mountain trek was not only inconvenient, it could be downright dangerous.

Steve was the poster child for not wanting to stop what he was doing because his body couldn't handle it anymore, but he also knew that the knowledge he had about how to train his body wasn't getting him where he wanted to be. He knew how to subject himself to physical and mental challenges like no one I had ever met, but that wasn't helping him fend off the limitations that were threatening to disrupt his ability to take on those challenges. So like Ruth, he decided I could help.

Ruth and Steve and I — and countless other clients and students thereafter — all became Unbreakable. And not because any of us were blessed with good luck or good genes (neither of these things makes an Unbreakable human, anyways). It also wasn't because we managed to avoid aches, pains, and setbacks.

We all experienced all three of those at various points along our journeys and all three will most certainly be present along your journey as well. How you handle these issues and learn from them says much more about your Unbreakable-ness than the fact that you experienced them.

You see, part of being a human who moves their body is accepting that sometimes your body is going to speak up and let you know that something needs attention. Becoming Unbreakable is not about eliminating any possibility of aches and injuries but rather operating from a place where the objectives are to live life fully, and when unexpected things pop up, you learn from them, tend to them, and become better because of them. With that being said, you *can* make yourself more resistant to aches and injuries, and you can become more resilient so that you bounce back from them better.

If you've ever had an injury that seemed to take forever to heal, or worse yet, never fully resolved, you already know how much time gets lost when aches and injuries overstay their welcome. Ruth, Steve, and the rest of my students and clients make themselves more resistant to aches and injuries by building what I call the Six Pillars of an Unbreakable Body.

The Six Pillars are a framework I developed to highlight important areas of care for your body. When you build these six areas up to have enough function, mobility, and strength, they will give you physical capacity and fitness that helps you feel your best and tackle all the activities you enjoy.

Through building their Six Pillars, both Ruth and Steve forged a strong base in their body upon which they could layer all the other sport-specific fitness they wanted to have so that they could go on every adventure and participate in each activity they loved, without hesitation that their body wouldn't support them.

Back then, I was in my first decade of becoming Unbreakable, and folks would frequently tell me, "Just wait until you're older." I'd point them to Ruth and Steve, who were the living example of what becoming Unbreakable could look like when you're older. They both had a strong attitude about becoming their unique vision of what Unbreakable looked and felt like to them. And they both were most certainly never going to let it be 'too late' to do the things they loved. They became Unbreakable, not because I gave them something they didn't have, but because they showed up with a desire that they wouldn't let die.

They brought me on board to support their journey with knowledge and expertise about training their body so it felt and moved how they wanted it to feel and move, and they adopted a mindset that allowed them to always be an active participant in the journey.

It's been 20 years of building and supporting my Unbreakable body and I'm still waiting for whatever it was those folks meant when they said to "wait until I'm older." In this time, not only has my body and my relationship to it changed, my entire life has changed. I know that sounds hyperbolic if you currently just want some relief for your joint pain — maybe you're not looking to change your whole life, and trust me, when I first started down this path, I wasn't thinking about anything beyond my body and what wasn't working for me, either.

But something funny happens when you start becoming Unbreakable. A shift happens. You start to understand that you'll be the one to decide when it's 'too late' (ie, never) and what's 'too complicated' (ie, nothing, it's just a matter of what you think is worth the time). You start to know that you know what's best for you. You start to take an inquisitive approach to listening and responding to your body. You get clear on your values for yourself and you exemplify them in how you take care of your body. You build a relationship with your body where you're always learning from the choices you make and how your body responds, rather than berating yourself or your body.

And when this shift happens, stuff starts to change — not just in your body but in how you approach life. You develop a deep knowing, and you have experience after experience to back it up, that you are an excellent caretaker of your body. You make the right choices for your body, and you're always listening and responding and caring for your body. In turn, you make the right choices for your life, too. You rewrite the relationship you have with your body and you end up rewriting the relationship you have with your life. You create a body you love to live in, and along with it you create a life you love to live.

It turns out that the process of learning to move, build, heal, and care for your body is one of the ripest fields for harvesting personal growth that you'll ever find.

CHAPTER 2:

So What Does Becoming Unbreakable Look & Feel Like?

T he first thing to know about becoming Unbreakable is that my vision of what it looks and feels like is going to be different from your vision. This is because our values and our vision for ourselves — while possibly similar in some aspects — are likely to be different in others. The second thing to know about becoming Unbreakable is that it's not an end-goal to achieve but rather a lifelong experience to have.

There will be times when you are closer to your vision of being Unbreakable, when you've got the whole thing flowing just as you envisioned, and there will be times when you're further away from that vision and you're tripped up by things you didn't expect or that you don't yet understand. The third thing to know about becoming Unbreakable is that the process you use to move closer to your vision of becoming Unbreakable is as much a part of being Unbreakable as the vision is. Your 'how' is as important as your 'what'.

As you read this book, you're going to learn how to put all of this into practice in your own life, but first, you need to start envisioning what the concept of 'becoming Unbreakable' looks and feels like to you.

Creating this vision will help you know what you're aiming for in a world where it's easy to look around and wonder if you should just be doing what you see everyone else doing. All you have to do is open an app on your phone and you can instantly see what your friends are striving for. You hear all sorts of people pontificating about what you 'should' be doing and how you should be living your life. It's easy to fall into thinking, "Wait, *is that* what I'm supposed to be striving for? *Is that* what I should be doing?" By creating your own vision of what Unbreakable looks and feels like to you, you'll have a picture in your mind that will keep you focused on what really matters to you individually.

Your vision will also serve as a waypoint to return to when you've veered off for a bit and want to find your way back. Your vision of what Unbreakable looks and feels like to you will help you cultivate strength, and not just the physical kind. There will be times when life asks a lot of you and you'll be able to lean on things you've developed during your physical training and body care practice — patience, stick-with-it-ness, knowing you can overcome an obstacle, staying focused, problem-solving, practicing forgiveness... I could go on. These non-physical strength skills are going to give you a wellspring to draw from the next time life asks you to be strong.

For me, being Unbreakable means knowing that I listen to my body first and foremost, that I know how to interpret what my body is telling me and that what I don't know, I can figure out. Being Unbreakable to me looks like freedom. It means being present, so whether I'm at my desk working or out in the mountains adventuring, I can be fully attentive and immersed in it because my body isn't aching and hurting. It means being resilient and independent. It means doing anything I choose because I'm not held back by limits. It feels like trusting my body, and knowing my body can trust me to take care of it. It feels like confidence, ease, joy, and not having to think about what I'm doing — just being me as I do the thing.

And as I mentioned earlier, becoming Unbreakable is not a destination to arrive at, a box to check off, or a certification to achieve and put in a drawer never to be looked at again. It's a lifelong practice of cultivating that vision for yourself in your daily actions, and knowing that if one day you pop your head up, take a look around, and realize you've drifted from your vision that you're only one action away from moving closer to it again.

So being Unbreakable, for me, is also about being tuned into my body and what it's telling me, responding when it lets me know my attention is needed for something, and not beating myself up if I realize that I've not been listening and responding as well as I'd like. It's about challenging myself to rise to new heights, but also practicing compassion with myself when my mind has an idea about where we should be but my body is telling me otherwise. And finally, being Unbreakable is about making everything, absolutely everything, on my path work *for me*.

To help you start envisioning what Unbreakable looks and feels like to you, here are some questions I'm inviting you to answer. Becoming Unbreakable often begins with body stuff, because aches, pains, injuries, fatigue, feeling fragile, and feeling old is often what is the most noticeable disruption to doing the things you want to do and feeling the way you want to feel. But becoming Unbreakable is never exclusively about body stuff.

By desiring to address the things that hurt and that hold you back, addressing them successfully, and then moving into the realm of being able to pursue your dreams, desires, and passions without those old limitations, you're building far more than your body. You're building confidence in yourself, a deep well of knowledge about your body, you're learning more about who you are, and you're naturally going to translate all of that into other arenas of your life.

When you create a body you love to live in, you'll also create a life you love to live. Since becoming Unbreakable does often begin with body stuff, let's start there and then expand outward:

- What is it about your body that isn't working for you?
- What aches, pains, weaknesses, or disruptions would you be thrilled to see go away?
- Are there things you wish your body could do or ways you wish it felt?
- If you've got aches, pains, or issues, how often do you give brain space to noticing them, thinking about them, and worrying about them? What would you do with that brain space if you didn't have to spend it that way?
- If your body feels like it's not holding up for you, what aren't you doing these days that you used to do? What would tomorrow be like if you could do one of those things again? What pursuits would you take up if you knew your body would hold up for you?
- If you've been under the stressful burden of feeling concerned, fearful, and worried about your body and what lies ahead for it, can you picture what it might feel like if that burden lifted even a little bit?
- If you've been trying to find solutions for your body's

aches and pains, how much has it cost you financially? Is there something else you'd like to do with that amount of money in the future?

- If you've been feeling like it's a constant fight with your body, and like you're your own worst enemy, can you imagine what it might be like to turn this relationship into a harmonious one full of trust and friendship?

- When you hear the words 'becoming Unbreakable', what images, sensations, feelings, or emotions come up for you?

Let these questions rattle around in your mind and see what comes up. I strongly encourage you to write this down in a journal or on a sheet of paper. Start with whatever comes to the top of your mind and get it down on paper. But don't put the paper away just yet. Like many creative brainstorming sessions you'll often dump the 'top of mind' items first and then feel as though you've run out of ideas. You haven't; you just need to give your mind a chance to go further.

To help yourself do so, go further into each word or sentiment you put down on paper. If being Unbreakable to you means "being strong", take it further! What does being strong do for you? To me, being strong is a part of being Unbreakable because it allows me to do anything I want — from yard work to mountain adventures. In addition, it allows me to do those things with confidence because I know my body will support me. You can see these things in my

Unbreakable vision that I shared with you earlier.

Once you've clarified your vision as best as you can right now, save it in a memorable place so you can revisit it in the future. Over time, you'll have revisions, additions, subtractions, and clarifications to make to it.

Your unique vision of what Unbreakable is to you is the most important thing to cultivate and hold firmly to, and while your vision can adapt and evolve over time, never let it go. There will most certainly be people — perhaps even your own inner critic every now and again — who will try to make you believe that you're being ridiculous in your pursuit of this vision. Your job is to ignore them and hold steady on your vision, as it will guide your direction and the choices you make about how to get where you want to go.

Throughout this book, we'll weave together information that's been gathered from science and research, as well as information that can only be gathered by you through the tools and frameworks in this book that will help you navigate the journey successfully. In doing so, you'll develop a profound understanding of how to build and maintain a body you love to live in.

Right now, you have the opportunity to change course — no matter how 'off the path' you are. To get relief from the aches, the pains, the fatigue, the weakness, the worry, the disruption of unpleasant aging. To create a body you love to live in. To avoid what's avoidable, and to be as ready as you can for what's not. To feel great and move well in your body, and subsequently feel great and move well through your life. To make yourself more resistant to future aches and pains, and more capable of bouncing back quickly when an injury does occur. And to do so in a way that doesn't rely on hammering yourself with harsh workouts or harsh words. To make yourself an expert of your own body and what it needs. To know, with certainty, that you know how to care for your body — even when you don't yet know what to do about a particular situation.

You have the opportunity to learn how to ebb and flow through life, making consistent progress with your body and enjoying the experience of living in it. To take a holistic approach to your body and life, and start seeing them as so much more than just a singular event or action that determines how your body or life go from this point forward. To take on the role of being an excellent caretaker of your body, and in turn, your life. This is what it is to become Unbreakable.

And it is the opportunity of a lifetime. Not simply because taking this opportunity means you get to live in a body that feels good and can do things, but because your whole life *will* change when you do the work to build your Unbreakable body.

If you're new on this path of becoming Unbreakable, it may seem like the distance is far from where you are now to where living in a body that feels how you want it to. But you've covered that distance before — as a newborn to a child to an adolescent, you made huge strides in the way you can move, how you can control your body, the mental connections you can make, and the skills you can acquire. And you'll use the same process your body used when you grew from a baby to a child to an adolescent to help your body now. You've done this before, and you can do it again. And lest you think that growing and learning is for kids, not adults, keep reading and you'll see that just isn't true. There's an old saying, "The best time to plant a tree is twenty years ago. The second best time is now." So would you like to become Unbreakable now, *or now?*

Here's where we take it from here: First, you'll learn about body ecosystems and why they do what they do. After that, you'll learn the mental model that will help you become an expert in building a body you love to live in. This is key because without it, you'll simply be waiting around for someone to tell you what to do when really, you're the expert in You. Once you have that groundwork laid down, then you're ready to explore the most significant conversations you're in with your body every day that highly influence how it feels to live in your body. Understanding these conversations means you can then engage in them, influence them, and use them to build your Unbreakable body. This book is full of guidance, some of it is right there for the taking while other items of guidance require you to engage with it, think on it, and experiment with it.

I believe in you, dear reader. Let's set off on the journey now.

CHAPTER 3:

Your Body Is An Ecosystem

I went to visit my friends, Robb and Nicki, out at their new house. They had warned me that we'd likely be catching up while doing yard work because there was much to be done at the new place. I love yard work so this didn't deter me at all. Sure enough, we spent part of the weekend working outside while we spent time together.

One of my jobs was to destroy the roots of the goat's head plants that had proliferated on the property. Goat's head plant is an invasive species that also goes by the name 'puncturevine'. And puncture you it will. Goat's head easily outcompetes other native plant species, which means it's quite difficult to sustain a diversity of native plants in its presence. Diversity is very important to any ecosystem being sustainable, as everything from wildlife to pollinators to microbes that live in the soil are impacted by the diversity or lack thereof. My friends wanted a diverse and harmonious ecosystem, not to mention a yard that was usable, and the excessive amounts of goat's head plants were a painful hurdle in the way of achieving that.

While I was pulling roots, a man arrived at the house. He was a soil expert and my friends had invited him out to get his help making a long-term care strategy for the soil. I stopped pulling roots and came to listen to him talk. What he shared was revolutionary to me.

The soil expert told us that the presence of the goat's head plants in the yard was a clue about the health of the soil. That is, the goat's head plant was there for a reason — it's a response to something. In this case, it was a response to the soil which was currently tolerating the proliferation of the invasive plant. You can have soil that doesn't tolerate the plant, but that wasn't what my friends had at that point.

The soil expert told us the ideal way to get rid of the goat's head was to make the soil such that it was inhospitable for the goat's head to grow. Not by using herbicides, not by chopping them out, but taking care of the soil so that the soil quality would make it impossible for the goat's head to proliferate there.

My friends stood to reap a big long-term gain if they chose to play the long game. If they could make a more robust ecosystem by improving the quality of the soil, they would create an ecosystem that supports a diverse array of plants and disallows the goat's head to take hold.

Not only would they have gotten rid of what they didn't want (goat's head plants), they'd have made it so they get more of what they do want (other plants, grasses, and pollinators) with less effort required to maintain harmony in their yard. My friends hadn't asked for a yard of goat's head plant, but they moved in to this house and that's what this house came with. Now it was up to them to formulate a strategy to bring up the health of the soil so that the natural outcome was no more thorny goat's head. What that soil expert was saying sounded exactly like how I view the journey to becoming Unbreakable.

In order for you to stop feeling like it's 'too late' and to start becoming your vision of Unbreakable, the first thing to do is to start seeing your body as an ecosystem and yourself as its caretaker. Ecosystems are dynamic entities that are always in flux. Even when they have periods of apparent consistency in how they are functioning and what they are cultivating, they are actually always responding and adapting accordingly to the ever-shifting environment. The same is true for your body.

Ecosystems are influenced by both internal and external factors. The same is true for your body. What flourishes in an ecosystem is a result of how that ecosystem is managed, worked with, and supported. Over time, some things will flourish while others will dwindle. And just because something dwindles now doesn't mean it will stay on that trajectory forever. The same is true for your body.

Ecosystems are perpetually responding to both subtle and significant influences on the ecosystem. The same is true for your body. This is why I find it strange that there's a firmly entrenched myth out there that it can be "too late for you, buckaroo" while you're still alive. If you're alive, that means your cells, tissues, organs, bones, systems, and mind, are capable of responding. And if they're capable of responding, they're capable of adapting, every day until your last.

Two characteristics used to describe an ecosystem are 'resistance' and 'resilience'. Resistance is the tendency of an ecosystem to remain close to its equilibrium state, despite a disturbance. And the speed at which it returns to its initial state after a disturbance, as well as how far it can be driven from its equilibrium state and still return, is called its resilience.

These two words nicely articulate two key attributes you can build into your own body. How much can your body tolerate (ie, how resistant are you) before succumbing to an injury, exhaustion, pain, or any of the other things you don't want? And how quickly does your body get back to one hundred percent after an injury (ie, how resilient are you)? If you tweak your low back every six months, you're not likely to feel very resistant. Same goes for if you feel like you're constantly getting hurt doing "basically nothing." And if you sprained an ankle twenty years ago and it's never been the same since, you probably don't feel very resilient. Nor would you feel resilient if, after that back injury last year, you've not been able to get back to regular life stuff, let alone workouts or sports.

Resistance. Resilience. Those two words are a palpable part of becoming Unbreakable — you can feel it and see it in your body when you build your resilience and your resistance to injuries. This is why becoming Unbreakable is about much more than just a laundry list of things you build your body to be able to do. When your body supports you, and you know it, you can sense it throughout your existence. It permeates everything.

In nature, things like wildfires occur and can have heartbreaking consequences, but they also are imperative to the growth and maintenance of the area. Amidst the destruction, wildfires catalyze growth and change. A wildfire is a disturbance to the ecosystem, and disturbances are an inherent — and vital — part of any ecosystem. The ecosystem is what it is because things disrupt it from time to time.

The same is true for your body. You are you because of what you go through, and how you operate in the future will be influenced by what you go through today. Your version of a wildfire might be an injury, an illness you have to deal with, low energy that keeps you from feeling effervescent about life, or any set of circumstances that causes disruption to you, your body, and the experience you have living in it.

You might also face things that aren't a 'wildfire' per se, but that are unpleasant outgrowths of something your current body ecosystem is responding to. What's your version of the goat's head plant? What's that thing (or *things*) that are keeping you from becoming Unbreakable?

Maybe it's that low back pain that seems to pop up as an issue once every six months or so. Or it might be a shoulder ache that was intermittent but has now become constant, so much so that you wake up with it each day. It may be a whole host of disruptive aches, pains, and weaknesses that are bothering you so much that it's disrupted your quality of life. Or it might be one or two things that are irritating, and sure it would be really nice to get rid of them finally, but you're just working around them for now and trying to keep moving.

It could be realizing you lack the requisite fitness or body capability to do the activities you want to do, whether that's yard work, a game of pickleball with your local team, or the marathon through the mountains that you've always dreamed of doing. It could simply be the feeling that you don't know what to do to change — even though you'd really like to make a change, it all just feels exhausting and hopeless. These responses are triggered by something your current ecosystem is experiencing. They're not what you envisioned for yourself and your options are similar to those of my friends with their yard: complain about it and try to avoid the issue, or do something about it.

If you're like most folks, you have done a little bit of complaining (which is perfectly normal!) and a little — or a lot — of 'doing something about it'. The real problem occurs when doing something doesn't seem to be doing anything. The issue comes back, it lessens but never goes away, or it just doesn't seem to respond at all to what you're doing. Or worse still, you make headway with the issue you're dealing with but then some other issue pops up. It doesn't have to be this way.

The Signal/Response Principle

Your body is always responding to the signals it receives. And that is the most hopeful thing I've ever come to realize. When you recognize that signals are always coming into your body, and your body will always respond to those signals, it means that you can *always* influence your body. That means it can't possibly be 'too late' to move towards your Unbreakable vision you have for yourself.

If your body is always responding, then even when you're not pleased with the responses, like aches, pains, fatigue, or any of the things that keep you from feeling Unbreakable, by knowing that the response is *in response* to something, you can work backwards, in a sense, to solve the issue. If you remember those equations you'd get in math class where they'd give you one part of the equation and the answer to the equation, and then you had to work backwards to find out what the other part of the equation was, this is like that.

This means that as long as you've got the willingness

to work the equation, it will never be 'too complicated' to figure out. In addition, if you find yourself in a situation that is beyond your control, what comes next is always influenced by you — to make the most of a bad situation, to grow from the place you are (even if that's not a place you ever intended to be), and to take what's here and make it work for you, regardless of how crummy the situation is. I call this pattern of your body's responses to signals the Signal/Response Principle.

All of the things that make up your body — from the tiny cells that make up the bones, joints, muscles and tissues of your body, the nerves that are constantly operating your organs, to your thoughts, feelings, and cognition — are constantly responding to signals that are occurring in both your outer and inner environments.

Everything you have ever done, not done, and will do are signals which your body ecosystem will respond to. The Signal/Response Principle is a simple, but powerful, principle that helps you take the first step (and every step thereafter) on your path to becoming Unbreakable.

It is the principle that guarantees that you can always make an impact on yourself, get stronger or more flexible, become more resistant to future injuries, improve your skill at the sport you are passionate about doing (even if you're 60 when you first pick up the sport), and feel more confident that you can absolutely take care of your body no matter what comes along.

Once you start thinking in signals and responses, you can use your Explorer's Mindset — a powerful systematic process that will help you ask better questions and take more action — to confidently solve the issues that come up with your body. We'll take a deep dive into the Explorer's Mindset over the next few chapters, but for now, know that when you start asking better questions, you become an active participant in the process of caretaking for your body ecosystem.

So what are signals to your body? There are too many to count, but here are a few to help you get started:

- Sunlight
- The way you sit in a chair
- The protein content in a food
- If you fall on pavement and scrape your skin so bad it bleeds
- How you breathe
- Putting a fork into a toddler's hand to get them to start using it
- Practicing a foreign language or a style of dance or a type of workout
- Being immobilized in a cast
- The shoulder you carry your bag or purse on
- Taking up woodworking or a job that requires repetitive movements.

The signals that come into your body tell your body a number of things about how it should respond. Just like there are countless signals, there are also countless responses. Here are just a few examples:

- Your shoulder's range of motion increasing or decreasing as time goes on
- Developing calluses on your palms
- Going from feeling tongue-tied as you practice speaking French to being able to navigate a simple conversation entirely in French at a Parisian cafe
- Forming a scab on your scrape
- Getting a suntan
- Your muscles getting stronger, or your muscles getting weaker.

You signal to your body every day about what it should maintain and what it should de-prioritize, what it should adapt to and what it should become less proficient at. Your body responds accordingly.

Are there complexities to each of these responses and what signals contribute to them occurring? Of course. But do you need to understand every component of the complexities to know that avoiding prolonged exposure to the sun is one way to avoid getting a sunburn? No. And do you need to fully understand the neurobiology of how a child develops fine motor control in order to teach them how to use a fork? Of course not. You *could* learn all the complexities of such things if they interest you enough to do so, but your ability to work with signals and responses is not dependent on you going that deep. As long as you are curious about how the signals and responses play out in your individual body, you'll start to be able to make meaningful changes.

The responses your body is making can be small — like subtle changes to your stature that mean decades from now, you will appear shorter and more rounded than you are today, despite not having noticed a marked 'shrinking' effect. The responses can be big and quite noticeable — things like swelling, heat, and bruising coming to an area where you've sustained an injury. Some responses happen automatically (or, we hope they do), platelets working to coagulate your blood around an open cut, for example. Others only happen intentionally — the increase in muscular strength that resistance training gives you when you repeatedly perform a particular exercise with increasingly heavier weights.

We even can see responses to unintentional signals in modern life — for example, childhood myopia, where you have difficulty seeing things that are further away, among American children has more than doubled over the last 50 years.[1] Worsening eyesight is often attributed to genetics or aging, but researchers at the USC Eye Institute at Keck Medicine of USC in collaboration with the National Institutes of Health (NIH), did a study that adds to a growing body of research showing that "too much screen time and not enough

1 Aldrich, M. (2016, January 22). Too much screen time is raising rate of childhood myopia [Blog post]. Retrieved from https://keck.usc.edu/too-much-screen-time-is-raising-rate-of-childhood-myopia/

sunlight are possible key contributors" — or signals — that are causing the eye to change how it functions and thereby create myopia.

Whether automatic, intentional, or unintentional, signals create responses. And responses are informative. Responses tell you that your body is responding to *something*, and you completely change the game once you recognize that this Signal/Response Principle is always switched to the 'on' position with your body. That means it's never too late to investigate the responses your body is making and explore what kinds of signals you could send to get your body to respond with more of what you want and less of what you don't.

This makes you the most powerful influencer that ever existed, not of social media followers but of yourself. And the act of exerting your influence begins with understanding that the Signal/Response Principle is always ready to work for you.

Signal In, Response Out

If you lifted a heavy object today, and then you lifted that same heavy object repeatedly over the course of a month, the weight would feel easier to lift as time went on. This is due to adaptations your body has made to become more proficient at handling the demands you are imposing on it.

You sent a signal to your body by picking up something heavy. By doing it repeatedly, and sending that signal repeatedly, your body responds to make you more proficient at picking the heavy thing up. The signals your body receives tell your tissues and the cells that make them up that they need to become more proficient at responding to that particular signal. And if you send specific signals frequently enough over a given period of time, your body's structures, all the way down to the cellular level, will adapt accordingly.

Picture how calluses form or dissipate on your hands. If you frequently use your hands to do things like building furniture, doing manual labor, lifting weights, or rock climbing, you'll form calluses on your hands. Calluses form because the skin on that particular part of your hand is consistently exposed to friction — for a long enough period of time that the skin cells of that area form a thicker layer, and that increases the amount of friction the area of skin can tolerate.

However, if there is too much friction or force too quickly on the skin, instead of a callus forming, the skin will blister or tear. When it comes to adaptations in your body, the specifics of the signal play a big role in the type of response that is created.

Now, the responses your body makes to the signals it receives are sometimes a very obvious one-to-one relationship, where one thing occurs and something else occurs in response. Most of us have fallen off bikes, tripped over a curb, or taken some kind of fall where we left part of our skin on the pavement. It's clear that the impact of skin on hard ground is the signal that led to your skin tearing in response and perhaps a bit of blood oozing out of the wound. Once that has happened, your body kicks into gear to begin the work of forming a scab.

I think it's safe to say that if you have a scabbed knee, you know what it's a response to. But quite often, things like joint pain, muscle weakness, an achy back, recurring injuries, or low energy don't show up as a one-to-one relationship.

And while the aging myths that abound certainly try to create a one-to-one relationship by correlating your bad back or sore knees to the fact that you're now 45 — as if your age alone is the explanation for your pain — it just doesn't work that way. Now, I'm not here to tell you that age 45 or 65 or 85 should be the same as age 25. It is not, but the fundamental tenets of your biology don't change so drastically that it's a lost cause once you're 40, or 50, or whatever age you've been told is 'old'.

As you'll soon see, you have an unbelievable amount of influence on your body, its composition, and its capabilities. And the sooner you understand signals, responses, and the unique way that they are operating in your body, the sooner you can begin to exert your influence — regardless of your age.

A Web Of Signals

You are a marvelously complex being that has an almost incomprehensible number of parts, systems, processes, chemical interactions, hormonal changes, and so on, all of which interact with each other every day. As you begin to tune in to the responses your body is making, let go of your grip on the notion that one thing caused the response you're experiencing (and if you could just figure out what that 'one thing' is, you could rid yourself of it forever). The odds are greater that there were several signals that contributed, rather than just one. Here are two examples to illustrate this.

Imagine you joined a group weightlifting class at the local gym. Your goal was to get in shape, and to your delight, that seems to be happening. You notice that your body's composition seems to be changing, and you feel better in your body. If you take the Signal/Response Principle as a tool for deciding what caused you to attain these results, you'd probably assume that the exercises you were doing in class were what got you these results. But there are a number of other signals and responses that are going on beyond the exercises themselves, any (or all) of which could also contribute to your body adapting.

By attending a group class, you're around other people and that might have boosted your serotonin and dopamine, which you then carry over into other areas of your life, thereby reducing your stress levels. Or, as you and the other class members formed a bond, your sense of responsibility and commitment may have deepened and that carried over into acting with greater commitment in other health habits. Or, the workouts may have helped you to exert enough energy that you feel more fatigued earlier in the evening, and you're now getting better and deeper sleep, which contributes to your blood sugar and hormones being more balanced. These responses are like a cascading waterfall, one thing setting off another thing, any or all of which can impact your body's composition and how you feel in your body.

Now imagine your back has been hurting for some time. You decide to try a yoga program that is marketed specifically for people with back pain. Within a week, you notice that your back pain has diminished significantly. Hooray!

So was it the yoga program that worked for you? Or was it that by doing the program every day that week you felt more empowered, even on a subconscious level, and that made you feel less worried, which caused you to relax the low-level tension you'd been carrying in your muscles?

Or was it that the program was relaxing in a way that you'd not experienced in a long time and that shifted you away from a rigid focus on your pain and allowed you to have a bigger expanse of awareness, thereby making the painful sensations smaller in comparison?

Or was it that the poses in the yoga program caused you to move your joints and muscles in a way that you wouldn't have tried on your own, and in doing so you increased circulation and muscle contractions in the area, causing you to feel the area differently? Any or all of these responses could have contributed to your back feeling better.

At all times, systems that are operating, actions are occurring, parts are moving, environments are changing, neurons are firing, and a multitude of other stuff is happening in your body. All of it influences the responses your body makes to the signals it's receiving. Even with the vast array of knowledge that's been gathered by curious researchers wanting to understand the science of humans and how we function, you can't reliably tease any one thing out of this web of interconnected systems and say, "This is exactly how this works, and you will for sure, without a doubt, every single time, get this particular response if you do this one thing."

Even though that's exactly how a lot of solutions are marketed, it's not actually how it works. So instead of thinking of signals and responses as static one-to-one pathways, think of them like a web with lots of interconnected parts.

If that's not what you wanted to hear — if you were hoping for "change this one thing and everything will be better" — hang with me. In a few chapters, I'm going to share with you some of the most impactful conversations you're having with your body every day, and how you can influence those conversations in a way that leads to more body responses you prefer. More importantly, I'm going to teach you how to figure out *anything* when it comes to your body. And that's key because while there are some fundamentals that every human is likely to benefit from implementing, the reality is that you're a unique individual and some of that stuff requires tinkering to make it work perfectly for you.

In addition, there are going to be things that show up in your individual life that are outside what most other people will be dealing with. You're going to need a way of figuring them out, otherwise you'll be stuck with body responses you don't like and no way of knowing what to do about them.

"But can't you just give me a manual of all the signals and all the responses?" If you're wishing for such a manual, I get it. Humans want certainty. We want assurances. We want to know that we'll get at least an equal amount back for the amount we 'paid in'. We want to understand what went wrong, fix it, and never let it happen again — especially when the problem is irritating, disruptive, and costly in terms of time, energy, or finances.

Unfortunately, with bodies, the only certainty is that you're here now and one day you won't be. But there is one thing you can become certain about, and it is that your body is always responding to the signals it receives.

Now, if you're ready to start taking care of your body ecosystem, you're probably wondering where to start. Like I said earlier, there are a whole bunch of signals you *could* send to your body but which ones *should* you send? And which ones should you send first? Well, there's no one-size-fits-all approach. In order to find answers to these questions and forge your path forward — and feel like you're not just stumbling around in the dark — you need a systematic process. For that, it's time to learn how to use a mental model called, The Explorer's Mindset.

PART TWO:
The Explorer's Mindset

CHAPTER 4:

Tuning In

Have you ever ignored signs and symptoms from your body? Have you ever felt resentful of your body for falling apart on you, for making you feel older than your age, or for causing you so much pain? Have you felt like you're trying really hard but your body is making it impossible for you? Or perhaps, you're not tuned in to your body at all and you don't notice symptoms until they're like a giant siren blaring at you to get your attention. If so, I can relate — the day I found myself being pushed in a wheelchair through an airport because I couldn't walk to my departure gate gave me those kinds of thoughts and feelings.

The symptoms first became noticeable to me as a

hamstring strain after a running workout one day. From that day on I felt the hamstring all the time, but instead of shifting gears to slow down or pull back on my usual activities, I thought, "Eh, it's just a strain, I'm strong enough to push through," and tried to keep up my normal routine of work-outs. It was only natural — I had an agenda and it did not include slowing down or stopping for an injury, or listening to anything my body was telling me.

A few weeks later, the hamstring pain had grown into a deep, constant, ache and I finally relented. "OK, fine, this is clearly an issue I need to do something about," I thought. As I pondered what I could do to deal with this irritating issue, the one thing I knew was that doing as much standing and moving around as I usually did wasn't going to fly anymore, so I started a game of "let's make a deal with myself." *If I do less of this one thing, then can I still do that other thing*. Anyone who has had an injury knows there's a sort of bargaining that often creeps in while you're recovering. It's normal, but you should probably question the quality of any deal you're making when you're in a compromised state, as when injured.

As time went on, I had to relent even further as the pain grew in magnitude. My deal-making with myself wasn't working. I was thoroughly disappointed with my body for being such a hassle. It was then that I left for my one-week vacation from work for the year. After a few days relaxing on the beach, my hamstring seemed like it hurt just a little bit less. I misread that as a sign that I was healed enough to run on the beach. Face, meet palm. Being tuned in to the subtle (and not so subtle) responses from my body was not a skill I had developed yet.

A day after the beach run, my hamstring was catching with every step I took, a sharp pain shooting down the back of my leg as I swung my leg forward to take a step. I tried to walk as best as I could, but the pain was excruciating. I couldn't bring myself to put any weight on that leg anymore, and since I was flying home that day, I was in trouble. I needed to get through the airport in order to make my flight… and I had no way to overcome the pain and get there under my own power. I ended up having to request one of those wheelchairs that airports have to assist travelers to their gates. Once home, I had to get crutches so I could stay off the leg for a while.

Leading up to that excruciatingly disruptive hamstring injury, my attitude toward my body and taking care of it was "I'll drag you along kicking and screaming if I have to." I wasn't listening to my inner self at all (you know, that part of you that speaks up softly from deep within you and is usually right). I imposed my will on my body, my body's preferences be damned. I valued achieving fitness objectives at the exclusion of listening to what my body was trying to tell me it needed.

At that time, I had a belief system, rooted in fear, that if I didn't keep the gas pedal pushed down firmly every day of my life, that I'd lose. Lose what? Results, progress, control, to name just a few. I was listening to my ego and its need to control things (exercise seemed to be a great way to control my body) even if I was getting hurt in the process.

I held ample amounts of resentment, judgement, and frustration towards my body and there certainly wasn't a 'same team' connection between me and my body. It was an adversarial relationship at best. Was that really the kind of experience I wanted to have living in my body?

Over the last few decades, I've seen just how many different ways a person can experience an unhappy relationship with their body. Some experience unhappiness as it relates to food, others experience it as it relates to body shape. Still others experience unhappiness by type-A-ing their way through life while their exhausted body drags along behind them. And of course, there's the unhappiness that shows up from feeling that your body is frail, that it's breaking down, that it's holding you back.

There are many ways to have a strained relationship with your body, and while it sure would be nice to just get the 'right exercises' to fix your issue, the right exercises alone aren't going to make you Unbreakable. You'll need to cultivate your mind and spirit as much as you cultivate your body.

And this isn't just some hippy-dippy message here. The Explorer's Mindset — the seeds of which were planted during that hamstring injury I experienced — is intended to help you figure out exactly what to do for your body *and* transform your experience of living in your body.

A mentor of mine, Dr. John Turner, who is the founding director of Turner Chiropractic & Rehab Center, saw how much I was fighting with my body and how it was affecting my wellbeing. He said, "Maybe you could take a break from the workouts and all the intensity in life for a bit. You can always pick it back up again if you decide it's better that way."

My face said it all: a totally blank, 'this does not compute' stare. I left that visit with him thinking I'd just go ahead and ignore that advice. Except, I couldn't stop that second bit of what he said from rattling around in my head. *I could pick it back up again if I chose to set it down for a bit.*

I remember thinking to myself, "Well, I know how to achieve this level of myself because I've done it before, so I guess if I did try what he's saying and it didn't work, I know how to get back to where I am right now... right?" Cautiously, I gave his suggestion a go.

I began to pull back on strenuous effort and started making room for things I would have never given time to previously. I started living differently, and without realizing it at first, I began creating a paradigm shift for myself.

It was terrifying. You might know the feeling if you've ever upended something that was so woven into your image of yourself, your life story, and how you view the world. It's a vulnerable place to be, questioning things about yourself that you had previously believed, firmly, to be true or false. Whether it's your job, your body, the sport you play, your place in your family, your personality or something about you, you start wondering, "Who am I, if I'm not wrapped up in that anymore?"

It was slow, almost imperceptible progress at first. But eventually I began to notice that my body was starting to feel better, and more broadly, *I* was starting to feel better. My energy increased, I felt more refreshed when I woke up each day, and I began to feel more capable of managing whatever came my way. My hamstring started to move onto a trajectory of healing. And even though I wasn't doing my usual workout routine, I wasn't turning into a blob of goo who was too weak, too slow, or too tired to do everything I wanted to in my daily life.

Even though I wasn't moving through life at the pace I'd been accustomed to, I was still getting everything done that I needed to. As time went on, it was like a snowball picking up speed rolling down a hill, the changes becoming more pronounced, more significant, and more wide-spread throughout my body and my life.

But it wasn't simply backing off the intensity that made these changes happen. When Dr. Turner offered the suggestion of taking a break, with the understanding that I could always pick it back up again, he was actually offering me an entirely new worldview I could adopt. And with that worldview came a new mindset, and with the mindset came new habits and practices, and from all of that, my entire experience of living in my body radically changed.

Instead of being overcome by emotions, frustrations, and judgements about my body, and instead of being surprised by some new ache or injury that seemed to pop up out of nowhere, I developed a way of tuning in to all the responses my body was creating. I figured out how to work with those responses to find the signals my body needed to make new responses that I preferred. I learned how to be a part of the process of caretaking rather than simply reacting to each thing as it popped up. This became what I now call the Explorer's Mindset. It's a tool that has helped many to become excellent caretakers of their body and blaze their unique path to becoming Unbreakable.

When you adopt an Explorer's Mindset, you learn and enhance how to tune into your body and what it's telling you with each response it makes. You develop an ability to sense how your body responds (subtly and not-so-subtly) to signals you send. Instead of only noticing when alarm bells are going off, you notice little changes along the way, which can help you to take action sooner to adjust the signals you're sending your body and in turn support your body through every ebb and flow.

This is of the utmost importance in a day and age when there is a lot of noise out there telling you what you should do and how you should be. In addition to becoming an expert at listening to your body, the Explorer's Mindset helps you figure out what the right actions are for *your* body and what it's telling you it needs. Instead of trying to fit yourself into the mold of what other people say is good to do, you take all those options and suss out which ones are *really* the good ones for you, which ones need to be altered in some way so they can be a good thing for you, and which ones just aren't good for you at all (even when some expert touts them as good.)

Instead of feeling at the mercy of some external force, whether that was 'aging', 'bad luck', 'bad genes', or someone else's opinion of how you should take care of your body, the Explorer's Mindset helps you learn that your body autonomy trumps all, that you are the one who is in charge here. You take your rightful place in the driver's seat of your body and life. Instead of failing to see the mental and emotional hurdles that show up on the path (and running smack into them), you'll develop the ability to recognize them and navigate your way over each one.

For me, adopting the Explorer's Mindset helped me figure out what actions to take to build my body so it would feel how I wanted it to feel, and so that it could do what I wanted it to do. It helped me figure out what additions and subtractions to make to my workouts and my daily routine so that both were truly tailored to my and my body's needs. It helped me figure out who to turn to for expertise I didn't have, so that I could accomplish something I didn't yet know how to do. And in the times I was dealing with an ache or a pain, it helped me squeeze the juice out of the experience so that I learned more about my own unique operating system and how to support it.

The Explorer's Mindset also helped me navigate my inner world of worries, fears, beliefs, and attitudes, and not just understand them better, but find an actionable way to root out the inner stuff that wasn't helping me, and replace it with something more helpful for me.

As I accumulated this kind of information about what my body needed, it made my decision-making process more effective and efficient and it made my selections of things to do or not do more automatic and intuitive. When I use the phrase "become an excellent caretaker of my body", this is what I'm talking about. Not some notion of excellence that equates to perfection, being the 'best', or being lucky that I don't have difficulties to contend with, but rather learning how to use tools that help me take everything on my path and put it to work *for me* to build my body, mind, and spirit to become Unbreakable.

Because it's not just achieving whatever end goal that is in mind that makes a person Unbreakable, remember, becoming Unbreakable isn't even a destination that once you've gotten there it's all done and dusted. Rather, it's a way of living, operating, and being a participant in the journey of your life.

Exploring A New Place

To begin with The Explorer's Mindset, imagine you've travelled somewhere far away and quite different from where you came from, and that other than you being here now, absolutely no one has ever been to, or resided in, this particular place before. It's your job to explore this place so you can learn about it, understand it, and to figure out how to use what's here so that it's a hospitable place for you to live. You need to understand the ecosystem, what makes things grow, what resources you can use, and which ones you'll need to put some effort into cultivating.

It's your first day in this place and you've begun your exploration by going out for a walk on a nearby hillside, and you're noticing details about it — how tall the grass is, what the air smells like, how wet or dry the dirt under your feet is. As you walk and take stock of your surroundings, you keep collecting more tidbits about this place — the types of plants you see, the shade of blue of the sky, and so on. Good job explorer, you're gathering a lot of helpful information about this new area!

Soon you'll start working with the data you're collecting, doing experiments with it to see how you can influence it, figuring out what you can do to get more of the good stuff that's already here, and what you might do to cultivate things you'd like to have but that aren't here in abundant supply. That's very important to do, since being able to live here in the future depends on you figuring out how this place works, what this place has, what it doesn't, and if you can influence that to make it as hospitable for you as possible.

You keep walking the hillside, but as you do, you feel judgements start welling up in you. You start shifting from, "This grass is tall and prickly," to "Stupid grass, you make my ankles itch." You begin to think that while the blue sky is *fine,* it really would be *better* if it had more clouds to cool you off from the hot sun. Your noticing shifts entirely into passing judgement about this place.

Before long, you're a big pile of judgements and anger and you can't focus on collecting the data about this place, let alone pondering which experiments you should start with — the two things that are your primary job as the explorer of this area, and which are required if you are to ever have a hospitable life here.

Now, you're probably thinking, "That's ridiculous, I would never get all worked up and judgey about something as benign as my surroundings." Well, now switch out 'a new place that you're exploring for the first time' with 'your body'. Your 'surroundings' are the body you're living in. You're the explorer of these surroundings, and it's your job to figure out how everything works here, as well as how to make it a hospitable existence living here. And remember, no one has ever been here before so it really is up to you to figure out everything about this place. Still true that you'd never let judgement, anger, betrayal or frustration, disrupt your exploration?

If you're like 99% of humans, the answer is 'probably not'. The Explorer's Mindset is about taking note of your body's ecosystem you're living in every day, learning about it, and trying out experiments with it to see if you can positively influence it to make it into the very best ecosystem you've ever lived in (because it will be the only one you ever live in.)

The process begins with realizing that every day you are collecting data about your body. The responses your body is always making to the signals it's receiving, those responses are data which tell you about your body ecosystem, and that informs you about what actions you can take to make the improvements you desire.

Whether you feel flexible, achy, strong, tired, or full of joint pain, whether the data is broad in scope — "every part of my body is just achy" — or extremely precise — "the inside corner of my right knee hurts every time I kneel down but is otherwise fine" — everything about how your body responds is data which you can use.

And when you process, interpret, and organize the data to make it meaningful and useful, it becomes information. You can use that information to make choices for yourself, to do experiments that communicate new signals to your body, to understand yourself better as you observe what kinds of responses your body makes to those signals, and to curate the responses that work best for you so as to make it a more hospitable existence in your body. In doing so, you'll turn that information into knowledge that you'll refer back to time and again to guide yourself forward to feeling and moving your best.

In time, that knowledge becomes deeply rooted, hard earned, well-curated, wisdom. And as you'll soon see, the three aspects of the Explorer's Mindset — 'explore, experiment, curate' — is the name of the life-long game of being a wise, excellent, caretaker of your Unbreakable body. Now, to make a place better, first, you must know the place. And so begin with the first component of the Explorer's Mindset: explore.

CHAPTER 5:

Go Exploring

Step one to being an explorer of your body is to take a good look at your current surroundings. Begin first with the inner world of your body: how it feels, what it can and can't do, what seems to be missing or not working. Then move to your outer world, which can include things like what your current work-life balance looks like, what's working well in your life and what's stressing you out, things you can do, things you can't do, and things you can only do with a struggle.

It might be tough to acknowledge and accept where you are right now if you've got stories in your head about where you should be. It will also be difficult to honor your true starting point if you're beating yourself up with 'should have's' because you dislike the current state of your being. For example, 'I should have taken better care of my body' or 'I shouldn't have kept pushing when I felt that tweak in my back'.

In addition, if you find yourself comparing anyone else's starting point to your own, or if you catch yourself trying to 'keep up with the Joneses' (a phrase that began in a financial/consumption sense and has since spilled over into body care, activities, diets, and more), it's going to be much more difficult to accept the reality of where you are today. It can also be challenging to truly accept the fact that making any sort of change takes time, and thus, you're going to need to be tolerant of your body and yourself as you live with things that you'd really like to see changed.

Just know that the current status of things is not the permanent status of things. And while you don't need to spend life navel-gazing, your process of exploring your inner and outer worlds will never end. Exploring is a way to collect data that you can put to use in the next two steps of the Explorer's Mindset — experiment and curate. Exploring is a way to notice what's changing, what's not, and to pick up on what's new to your awareness. That is, you're not likely to tune in to every single thing that your body is responding to, but over time you'll likely notice some things that you can clearly tell you did not notice before.

Here are a few categories of responses you might collect data in, relative to exploring your body (though you're certainly not limited to these nor should you feel as though you have to collect data in all of them):

- How your body feels in a broad sense of assessment: "my joints feel really achy today"
- How your body feels in a more specific sense of assessment: "my hip hurts, especially by my butt cheek, and it feels more like a deep ache than a surface-level one"
- How your body feels before/during/after certain activities: "my back feels tight after having been in the car for an hour commuting to work"
- How your energy levels feel to you: "I feel like I need a nap every day around 3pm"
- How your temperament feels to you: "I've been feeling grumpy and short-tempered"
- How certain foods make you feel: "I feel really energized after eating that meal"
- How certain people make you feel: "I feel so good spending time with that friend"
- How the reps of an exercise in your workout felt: "ten reps felt hard"
- What your general movement throughout the day seems to be like: "I sit a lot"
- How you do a particular movement in your day: "I noticed that when I hold my child, I always shrug up my shoulder into my ear and push my hip out to one side"

- What that painful sensation you've been noticing in your hip lately is feeling like today: "it's throbbing today and it wasn't throbbing yesterday"
- What your outer world is full of lately: "work has been nuts, my sleep has been terrible, and I'm worried about my sister and the struggles she's going through right now"

Keep in mind, your data collection need not be predominantly for things you don't prefer, though that tends to be what someone notices first and most in the beginning. Becoming aware of when you appreciate, value, are proud of, and grateful for, how your body felt, moved, or supported you, is as much a part of making life in your body hospitable for you as improving things you don't like.

As you collect your data, it's highly likely that there will be some stories and emotions tethered to it. In those stories you're likely to find things like self-judgement, comparison, worry, blame, resentment, other people's opinions, and so on. This is totally normal, and in fact, it's so common to tether data to stories or emotions that you might not even realize you do it.

Here are some examples of stories and emotions tethered to data:

- My hip hurts (data) *and I'm worried I will be in pain forever* (emotion about the data).
- Ten reps felt hard (data)... *everyone else can already*

do this easily, I'm failing (story about the data).

- Ugh, my shoulder's acting up again (data), *what did I do wrong this time?!* (story about the data).

Notice the distinct difference between the body response, and the stories and emotions that are about the body response.

Humans naturally attach meaning to things. It can be very helpful for making sense of a situation. And experiencing emotion is quite natural as well; in fact, it seems to be far more connected to decision-making than you might at first realize.[2] Emotions and stories can also be excellent catalysts for change. They serve as good reminders of what you want to feel more of and less of. They can be a useful tool through which to learn so much more about yourself, and they're as much a part of the Signal/Response Principle as the data you're collecting about the physical responses your body is making.

For instance, if you struggle to trust your body because, as you see it, it's failed you so many times that it doesn't deserve your trust, that's a fair response. Think about the last time you had to interact with someone you didn't trust. Was it easy or difficult to be fully relaxed and invested in the interaction with that person? If that experience feels familiar in terms of how you deal with yourself, make a mental note

---

2 Lerner, Li, Valdesolo, and Kassam (2014 September 22). Citation: Emotion and Decision Making. *Annual Review of Psychology*, 802. Retrieved from https://scholar.harvard.edu/sites/scholar.harvard.edu/files/jenniferlerner/files/emotion-and-decision-making.pdf?m=1450899163

of it, as this could be ripe terrain for experiments.

Or if you feel that parts of your body are the worst because they hurt or feel weak, your opinion is understandable. Now think about a person you've formed a negative opinion about and how that has influenced your ability to see them in any other light. Here again, if this sounds like how you think of yourself, experiments on this may be of value to you.

What if you've disconnected from parts of your body out of fear, frustration, or because they've been a source of stress? That's fair. Imagine a loved one was going through a difficult time. Would you encourage them to numb out to the situation to avoid dealing with it, or would you want to help and support them as they go through it and come out the other side? Once again, if this resonates, you may have found something worth experimenting on.

As you investigate your own stories and emotions, you'll find that each one is there for some reason or another, but when these stories and emotions stick around longer than they're useful, when they don't get questioned about their validity, and when they override other more tangible data that could help you make the next decision you need to make, they need to be checked.

Just as you can send new signals to get new body responses, so too can you send new signals to write new stories and tend to your emotions to make them work in a new way for you. The questioning framework we'll work through next will help you check those stories and emotions.

But first, have you noticed just how often the stories and emotions you have about your body are negative? I believe there are a few key reasons for this: negativity bias, long-standing common narratives that the older you get the more of a problem your body is, and lack of practice in writing alternative narratives.

A negativity bias is the notion that things that you deem negative or unpleasant stick out more to you and influence your behavior more than things you deem positive. If your low back is sore today, you're likely to notice that far more than you notice other positive things your body has experienced today. And while it's helpful that your brain is always scanning the environment for potential threats, it can become a hindrance in making tangible forward progress if it becomes your dominant worldview.

Unfortunately, it's incredibly difficult to check your negativity bias when the narrative you hear most commonly is that bodies are a problem. I don't think anyone sets out to pass that notion along to anyone else, but it's pervasive in the messaging you've likely heard, both as you were growing up and now.

Even if no one has ever said that to you directly, there's copious amounts of marketing messages in advertising that perpetuate the narrative. "Your body's got a problem... solve your problem by buying this thing!"

As we've seen, it's also common to hear that age correlates

to how you should expect to feel — "At your age, of course your knees are going to hurt." The implication is clear, as you age your body becomes a problem. I've met people of all age ranges, from 35 to 65, who told me they were told that they should probably cut back on the activities they love or they should just expect their body to feel achy or broken. How ridiculous! Who decided that bodies just feel bad as they get older? Who decided that the narrative we're going to go with as a society is that you are a prisoner of your body? That is an incredibly restrictive viewpoint on bodies, as if a body is a ball and chain you are stuck with.

If you feel like someone or something is placing restrictions on you that you didn't ask for and don't want, it's only natural to resent the person or thing that has put those restrictions on you — in this case, your body. Now, if you've grown up hearing this kind of narrative, and you've had decades of practice feeling frustrated by your body, it's understandable that you're not well-practiced at writing an alternative narrative for your body and the experience of living in it.

But the good news is that you've already started to write a new narrative when you crafted your vision of what becoming Unbreakable looks and feels like to you. And as you learn how to use your Explorer's Mindset to make life in this body ecosystem of yours as hospitable as possible, you're going to continue writing a new narrative for yourself.

As you collect your data, take stock of both the physical responses you're noticing, and the responses that are more in the realm of judgements, worries, stories, beliefs, or fears. A key component of the Explorer's Mindset is making everything work in your favor in some way. Your data about physical responses you're experiencing will be a central hub of action for you as use your Explorer's Mindset to do the things you likely think of when you think about 'building your body' — incorporating movement, trying various forms of exercise, cultivating new daily activities, exploring habit changes, and so on.

But the cultivation of your Unbreakable vision for yourself won't be exclusive to just the physical activities you do for your body. The non-physical stuff like stories and emotions are going to give you as much growth as any exercise or training program will for your muscles and joints.

Remember, becoming Unbreakable is not just a feat of strength or flexibility. It's going on the journey of a lifetime, choosing a way of living, and taking care of the You that inhabits your body as well as caring for the physical structures of your body. Becoming Unbreakable is about the substantial, varied, unique, and soulful experience of learning how to speak the same language as your body, developing deep wisdom about your body, building your autonomy, and finding joy in the experience of living in this body of yours. And every single thing you discover as you explore your body ecosystem is valuable for getting you there.

Curious Compassion

You already know that the point of exploring is to do so without judgement and frustration. But if you've never taken stock of your body ecosystem's current environment with anything other than resentment and irritation, you might not know how to take stock without them.

One of the cornerstone skills the Explorer's Mindset develops within you is what I call *curious compassion*. As you collect your data, curious compassion allows you to move from an exasperated "ugh" to an inquisitive "huh" — as in, "huh, that's interesting."

By tapping into curious compassion, you're able to perceive something in your body — especially something you don't prefer like an ache or a pain — and wonder what the sensation is all about, rather than begrudging it. When you explore and collect data using curious compassion, you're able to start moving away from thoughts like, "Of course my stupid body hurts again", and towards thoughts like "Well, I know my body isn't trying to make me miserable, so let me explore what's going on here."

It's totally fine to feel frustrated and to sulk about something for a bit, but at some point you have to shift into action mode, and stewing in frustration or disappointment is only going to make it harder to do so. Curious compassion helps you see that your body is not trying to hurt you, it's not intentionally setting out to make your life difficult, and it's not cursed or irreparable. It's just being a body that is doing body things, and how it's responding is helpful information that you'll be able to use.

Think about the last time you noticed symptoms that indicated you might be fighting off a cold. Perhaps your head started feeling stuffy, your body felt tired and achy, and you got a bit of a chill.

At first, you might notice those symptoms and think, "Ugh, I don't have time for this!" You can ignore the responses your body is making, keep on keepin' on, and you might make it through just fine... or your symptoms will increase and you'll be forced to take a rest day or three. Alternatively, you can use those kinds of immune-response symptoms to adjust course to give yourself a bit of extra rest and recovery. Perhaps you get an extra hour of sleep that night, call off your workout for that day, or go home to take a hot shower and rest on the couch for a bit. You might still end up whammied by the virus for a few days, but you might also create just enough space in your body's ability to respond that you don't feel the effects of the immune response as much, and you're back to one hundred percent faster.

Whether it's symptoms of an immune response to a virus or a subtle ache in your knees during a workout, exploring and collecting data with curious compassion helps you hear the conversation that's coming from your body and helps you come up with ways to adjust course. One of my students shared an example that demonstrates this nicely:

"I was in my second set of squats and felt a funny little tweak in my knee. In the past, I'd have ignored it because I cared more about being able to say I completed the workout as it was written than I did about if my body was feeling capable of completing the workout.

I took my rest break to move around a bit with my knee and see if I felt OK to try my next set of squats. It wasn't like it felt injured, but it didn't feel stellar. I thought about my options, which before would have been a grand total of two: keep going, or stop. But learning to use my Explorer's Mindset helped me to see that I actually have more options — I could do a lighter weight, I could try a different exercise instead of the squats, I could go on to other exercises and try the squats again later, and I could even decide to just skip the rest of the sets that day because it doesn't mean anything about whether I'm successful or not.

So I tried out a step-up exercise instead and my knee didn't bother me at all, so I did the rest of my sets as step-ups instead. In the past, I've ignored little tweaky stuff like that, and I've definitely had it become a big problem because I just pushed through it.

That usually led to having to take time off my workouts, which meant I lost progress and momentum, which made me feel awful and like I was starting over. Now I know, making little shifts and adjustments as I listen to my body is how I keep making forward progress. The Explorer's Mindset really clarified that for me."

It's true: whether you're supporting your immune system as it fends off a cold or adjusting your workout mid-session based on how you're feeling and moving through each repetition, you'll keep the forward motion going if you ebb and flow with your body more than if you drive forward regardless of what your body is telling you it needs.

The path to anything in life — including becoming Unbreakable — is never a truly straight line. When you have a mental picture about how your path *should* look and feel, anything that doesn't match the picture in your mind will feel wrong or bad. But if you can set your mind on the fact that curves and swirls are actually how 'doing it correctly' looks and feels, and thus, you're never off track, you'll not only feel better about the whole thing, but you'll also learn more as you move along the path. And if it looks like someone else's path was a simple, straight, line, the reality is that you just aren't close enough to see all the loops, swirls, and circling back that occurred in their journey.

Now, here's where folks tend to get tripped up: thinking that they won't make forward progress if they don't hold the standard of pushing hard through the body's discomforts. But there is a difference between the discomfort of *effort* and the aches or pains that indicate your body needs something other than what it's getting. The only way to differentiate between them is to become proficient in the language of your body.

Unfortunately, it might be difficult to understand the language when you first start. If you have learned to ignore any part of your experience, you may need to practice tuning into your inner and outer surroundings. If you were told that things with your body are predominantly influenced by aging, you may need to learn how to widen the lens through which you view your body. And, if you've simply never listened to your body for whatever reason, it will take time to build up to being a good listener.

Using curious compassion as you explore and collect data is a result of taking an eyes-open, full-frontal view of what it's like right now to live life with your body. No hiding from stuff you don't like, no ignoring stuff your body desperately wants you to pay attention to, no shaming yourself for past choices that brought you outcomes you don't prefer. Just accepting it all, taking a deep breath, saying "I've got this", and moving forward as such into the next aspect of the Explorer's Mindset: experiment.

CHAPTER 6:

Preparing Your Experiment

It was a fun, dynamic, rock climbing problem that had a jumping move where you go from one set of small rock holds to a big ledge by jumping up and out to the right. I had done it successfully several times and I just wanted to do it one more time before my friends and I wrapped up our climb.

I jumped, grabbed the big ledge between my fingers, felt my feet swing out to the side just like the last time — but unlike the last time, I felt my fingers slipping off the ledge. In half a second I was airborne, then my feet grazed the ground, my knees buckled to the right, and as I landed I heard a pop. I crumpled to the ground pulling my knee to my chest, the pop sound making it all but certain that I'd just done significant structural damage to my knee. I couldn't believe it. I'd ruptured my ACL.

Falling is a part of rock climbing, and I knew how to fall safely. But this fall was unexpected and I hadn't been ready for the landing. You try to avoid situations like this, but sometimes it just happens.

The force of my bodyweight, plus gravity, plus momentum, meant that the anterior cruciate ligament of my knee had torn, and knowing what goes into ACL rehab, as soon as I heard the pop I knew I was about to spend months hobbling about, doing rehab work I didn't want to do and *not* doing fun things like skiing, snowshoeing, and climbing. Damn.

Instead of spending the next several months building my body for adventurous pursuits as planned, I would be having a long and continuous conversation with my body's tissues to regain motion and support in my knee, and to rebuild the strength and capacity of my leg.

My Unbreakable vision for myself did not include 'heal myself from an ACL rupture.' But due to this unexpected event, it was added to my vision for me, and I could either take it on and work on it with as much motivation as I'd been working on my original vision, or I could accept my bad luck and let it dictate the rest of my life for me.

I chose the former, and thanks to all of the lessons I'd learned in the decade or so since that hamstring injury, the healing process — while painful and difficult — went more smoothly, effectively, and believe it or not, happily.

Once you've begun exploring and collecting data about your body ecosystem, it's time to start taking action with experiments. Experiments are how you send specific, intentional communication to your body, by way of an action, and how your body responds is the result of the experiment. From there, you're able to identify communication that is worth sending consistently and over time, you can curate your personal method for building and maintaining your Unbreakable body.

With my ACL in tatters, that evening I settled into life on the couch, my leg propped up amidst a mountain of pillows. After testing a variety of positions and pillow configurations, I found one that made the throbbing less severe, which made it possible for me to get to sleep. The next morning, I got up to a sitting position on the couch and began contracting my thigh muscles, then my calf muscles, then attempting to gently move my toes, feet, ankles, knees, testing what triggered pain.

A lot of movements hurt, but some didn't. Once I knew where the points of pain were, I stayed away from those areas and proceeded to do joint movements and muscle contractions in all of the pain-free positions and ranges of motion every hour for the duration of my waking hours. As I did so over the weeks and months that followed, I paid attention to what kind of response my body's tissues made. The response was just that the muscles were working and my range of motion I could access without pain was increasing, and so I kept up those muscle contractions and movements.

The first week after the injury, I borrowed a friend's crutches to go out and do some errands, and while out I tested if I could put any weight on my injured leg while the crutches held the rest of my weight. I did one length of the parking lot with just a little bit of weight on the leg, and that was enough to tell me I shouldn't do that again anytime soon.

In the months that followed, not a day went by where I wasn't experimenting with my body, testing out movements and positions and muscle contractions to see what kinds of responses my body gave to them, testing my current limits.

"Can I stand on my injured leg to put on my sock on the other foot yet?" For a long time, the answer was "No, not yet." I noticed that a stressful week of work made the pain feel worse, and tested out ways to mitigate that. With each experiment, I was paying attention to the responses my body created and I used that as helpful data to guide each next action I took.

Now that we've covered how to start exploring, let's look at the process of doing experiments. The process of experimenting isn't a new idea. How else do you think our ancestors figured out which plants, when consumed, would kill you outright and which ones would make a flavorful gin? Truly, exploring and experimenting are how we gain knowledge about any and every subject. But when it comes to doing experiments specifically to improve the experience of living in your body, it's incredibly common to feel more like you're taking a stab in the dark.

And if you're like most folks, you weren't taught much when you were younger about how to care for your body, and so it feels difficult to know which knobs to turn and levers to pull. Sure, maybe you lucked out and had a parent who was into health or fitness in some way, but the rest of us likely had our only exposure to physical training and body care in grade school gym class.

And if you were lucky enough to even have gym class as a kid, you were luckier still if it wasn't 90% kickball and 10% 'health' class where you learned the correct names for sex organs. Not exactly helpful for knowing how to get from here to your Unbreakable vision you have for yourself.

The Unbreakable Field Journal

To figure out what your body ecosystem needs to become Unbreakable, it helps tremendously to have a structured process for doing experiments with the data you've collected. A good process for experimenting helps you organize, prioritize, and execute on the actions you think will help you move toward the Unbreakable vision you have. And as you do so, you'll gather invaluable wisdom about what your body needs to be Unbreakable.

Which is why I am going to strongly encourage you to store them in your own 'How To Be Unbreakable' field journal.

Keeping track of what you learn as you experiment is is beneficial for several reasons. One, you're a human with a life and that life probably has a lot going on in it. You're not expected to memorize all the signals you've tried and how your body responds to them.

Two, there are going to be times when the situation you're in doesn't happen all that frequently, such as with a more serious and disruptive injury or illness. If the last time you had something majorly disruptive to tend to was a decade ago, are you going to remember exactly what you did that worked well for you back then?

And finally, if you're not feeling tip-top because of some body response you're dealing with, anything to get some relief would be nice. If you can recall that doing a particular set of movements, or drinking a cup of a particular herbal tea, or going out on a short walk in the sunshine helped you feel just a little bit better the last time you dealt with something like this, then the quicker you can start moving towards relief.

You can use a simple notebook for this, or you can get the How To Be Unbreakable Field Journal I've put together as a companion to this book. Each page of the How To Be Unbreakable Field Journal is made to make it easy for you to track the most important information as you go on this journey of curating your unique protocol of what moves you towards your vision of what becoming Unbreakable looks and feels like for you. The journal contains pre-made record sheets to guide you through experiments and ensure you capture all the important information from your experiment, plus guided pages to assist you in tracking your Unbreakable vision and your body ecosystem over time, along with many other pages made especially to help you curate exactly what your body needs to be Unbreakable. Simply head to the book bonus page to pick up your copy: wwww.theunbreakablebody.com/book-bonus

Once you've considered how you'll track your experiments, it's time to go through the systematic process of doing a great experiment and gleaning helpful information from it. With the method of experimentation I'm going to teach you, which begins with four simple questions, you'll be able to navigate your way to the heart of every matter you're dealing with in your body. It gives you clarity on which experiments to do, and it also acts a lot like a friend with whom you can talk through a problem.

If you've ever been worked up about a situation and called a friend to talk about it, you know that simply by talking and feeling heard, you go from feeling like a messy mix of emotions and cluttered thoughts to feeling calm and rational again. In this framework, *you* are the friend you're talking to, and you're the one helping yourself move into that calmer place where you can start to take action.

The first step to doing experiments is deciding what you want to experiment on. You collected data about physical sensations you're experiencing as well as non-physical things like stories and emotions that seemed to be tethered to the data. From that group of data, pick something you'd like to try and influence.

What, What, What, Who?

There's a meme that goes something like this. The person is wondering why they don't feel good. Their brain answers, telling them to stop treating coffee like a food group. It then tells them to eat a vegetable and to get more sleep. The person replies with a shrug, and says, "I guess we'll never know!", to which the brain replies with an exasperated "Oh my god!!"

This meme illustrates the reality of trying to figure out what your body needs. There are so many things you can do that you can end up with analysis paralysis if you don't have tools to help you sort through it all. It's why I developed the 'Three What's & A Who' questioning framework.

Here are the questions in the framework, and then we'll go dive into each one specifically:

What external signals may have contributed to the response I'm experiencing?
What internal signals may have contributed to the response I'm experiencing?
What is the opportunity here?
Who can help?

'What' x 2

The goal with the first two 'What' questions is to help you identify possible signals in your current ecosystem, both outer and inner, that may be influencing the response you're experiencing. Remember that the Signal/Response Principle is always on, so the things you're experiencing are in response to *something*.

The response you made note of in your data collection could be a response to a singular signal, or a web of signals. By taking stock of possible signals, you can begin putting the experiment together because those signals will be what guides your experiment.

External signals include everything outside of you:

- The shoes or clothes you wear
- The way you're sitting in your desk chair
- How you're carrying your child on your hip
- Situations that are causing you to feel stressed (like having a job that isn't going well)
- Your sleep quality, and so on.

Internal signals are all the things going on inside of you and can include:

- How your muscles and joints are moving
- How much strength and mobility they have
- The tissue quality of your joint capsules
- Your level of balance and coordination

- How much inflammation your body is dealing with
- What your nervous system is responding to (like a stressful job situation)
- Plus other aspects of health such as blood sugar levels, how hydrated you are, your hormone levels, and so on.
- Internal signals can also include things you may not be able to quantify but you can sense, like how safe your body feels or if you're feeling anxious.

So ask yourself: what external or internal signal might have contributed to me experiencing this body response I want to change or improve? Make a list of the web of signals that could be influencing the response you've noted. It could be one of those signals working alone, or the combo of many signals creating this response. For now, just list them out.

These first questions also help you to gain context for the data you've collected, which help you understand the environment from which that response is coming. That's important because without context, you can end up wildly off-base in the way in which you tackle your experiment.

Imagine if you told a friend your foot was hurting and before you could say anything more, they responded with "Well, maybe take your shoes off and put your feet up." Seems reasonable enough, except that the reason your foot is hurting is because you just stepped on a nail and it's embedded in your foot. Taking off your shoes and putting your feet up probably isn't going to make the pain go away in this instance, but without any context, your friend was just giving advice that seemed reasonable given the information they had.

If that one seems far-fetched for you because you're hoping to never get a nail embedded in your foot, here's a more realistic example of why context is so important for the data you're collecting.

Imagine you're experiencing pain in your low back area, and you tell a practitioner, "My low back hurts", in the hopes that they'll tell you the solution to fixing the pain. Without gathering context by way of asking questions (exploring) to collect data, you and that practitioner are just guessing at what might be contributing to you feeling back pain. To illustrate this, let's look at just a few of the possible causes of pain in the low back:

- Muscles that are rigid and unable to contract and lengthen much beyond one particular position. (The question of *why* they are rigid in the first place is a whole other ball of wax that we'll dive into later, but it's relevant here too because not all rigidity is due to a muscle needing to be stretched more.)
- Muscles that are too weak for the demand that was placed on them
- A spine injury, such as nerve compression
- A kidney infection. Yes, kidney infections cause what feels like low back pain.
- Traumatic injury, such as taking a fall, being hit hard by

an athlete in a sporting event, or being in a car accident
- Tumors
- Pregnancy
- Menstrual cramps

If you and the practitioner don't examine the environment this response is emanating from, your guess about how to treat the pain could be wildly off-base.

By identifying the possible external and internal signals that may be contributing to the response you're experiencing, you're able to clarify a number of possible options for experimentation and by looking at your full list of signals you can prioritize which you should experiment on first.

Right now, you're not trying to find a definitive reason *for* your data but rather to help give a more detailed picture *about* the data. The experiment you'll do next is where you'll figure out more definitive answers, but right now, you're just gathering ideas so that you can choose one to experiment on first.

Now, you might be thinking right off the bat, "But I don't know about these sorts of things!" My dear explorer, this is a time that is ripe for exploring. If you don't know what external or internal signals may contribute to the response of aches, pains, or other body sensations you're experiencing, you can find out. Remember, you're an explorer, not an 'I-already-know-er'.

Read books, scour the web, work with a practitioner in the field that seems relevant to your query. Humans have been figuring things out since the dawn of time, and you are as capable as those earliest humans were. Here's an example of how you might start deciphering which internal and external signals you're experiencing and what they could mean for the response you are working on.

Imagine your hip feels stiff and achy, and it's been that way for a month now. You could start by reflecting on your history with your hips, any injuries or situations — however far in the past they may be — that might be related to what you're experiencing now.

Then you could shift to looking through your day and making note of the motions and positions your hips go through in a day. After that, you can reflect on your lifestyle, including what types of shoes and clothes you wear, your diet, your sleep, and your stress level.

Next, you could look at the internal signals… Are your muscles strong through regular weightlifting or some other form of activity that requires you to undergo regular strain? Do you notice your hip mobility has changed over the last few months or years? Are you feeling less coordinated in your motions lately? Have you started or stopped doing anything in particular?

These are just a few of the many signals you could examine to help you answer those first two 'What' questions. You can also do research yourself to learn about signals you may not have as much knowledge on yet by looking things up online, picking up a book on the subject in question, or talking with professionals who are experts in the field you're exploring. Of course, you'll want to take a mindful and measured approach to consuming information; even research papers can be skewed towards the outcome desired by whomever is paying for the research. Good questions to ask yourself as you gather information: *Who is the source? Is anyone else saying something similar? What might they be overlooking? Does this seem reasonable? Is my bias influencing how I view this? What assumptions might they be working from that might actually not be true?*

A healthy dose of skepticism is useful when learning. It is actually a byproduct of curiosity, so it's not a bad thing so long as it doesn't stop you from taking action. (We all know the person who is so skeptical of everything that they never try anything. That's not healthy or productive skepticism.) In addition to not letting unhealthy skepticism stop you, do not be stopped simply because you fear getting the answer wrong. It's completely normal to be wrong sometimes, and the sooner you accept that, the sooner you can take that next action step. Besides, the right answer is to *take action*, which you are, thus you got it right.

Your answers to these first two questions will become more nuanced the longer you use your Explorer's Mindset. The more experiments you do and the longer you cultivate your body ecosystem, the more you'll learn. And all of that learning will become wisdom which will help you see things and select things you wouldn't have before, when you didn't have as much information and experience to lean on.

Whether it's figuring out foot pain, sussing out a symptomatic shoulder, learning how to get physically strong for the life you desire to lead, or re-writing a story you have about your body and how it can't be trusted, whatever you take on to try and make life in this body of yours as hospitable as possible will give you a bounty of wisdom you'll be able to lean on again in the future.

One More 'What'

Now that you've answered the first two 'What' questions, it's time to go to the third one: *'what is the opportunity?'* Instead of seeing the issue you're dealing with and all the possible signals that could influence it as exasperating problems, start seeing them as opportunities. With my coaching clients, we've long referred to things they are dealing with in their body as "areas of opportunity", rather than problems. Instead of "this is my bad hip", it's "my right hip is one of my areas of opportunity." Think it's just a game of semantics? Here's the definitions for both words:

> **Problem:** 1. A question raised for inquiry, consideration, or solution 2. An intricate unsettled question; a source of perplexity, distress, or vexation; difficulty in understanding or accepting.[3]

3   Merriam-Webster. (n.d.) Problem. In *Merriam-Webster.com dictionary*. Retrieved October 1 2020, from https://www.merriam-webster.com/dictionary/problem

Opportunity: 1. A favorable juncture of circumstances, 2. A good chance for advancement or progress.[4]

By seeing things as opportunities rather than as problems, you'll naturally shift how you view your body, your efforts, and your outcomes. When you view your body as a problem to be solved, you're far more likely to think in a narrow and rigid frame of mind, and you're more likely to increase the amount of effort, strain, and frustration that bubbles up as you try and solve said problem.

As the definition mentions, you're more likely to see it as a source of stress. In addition, your brain will always take the path of least resistance to find an answer, and you'll narrow the path of least resistance even further when you're under stress. In an article titled, 'Understanding the neuroscience that fuels creative thinking can make you more innovative', neuroscientist Dr. David Eagleman says: "In order to proliferate options, our brains need to get off the path of least resistance and reach more widely into its networks. This means not settling for the first solution that comes to mind, but constantly searching for more."[5]

That means the first idea that comes to you to solve the current situation is unlikely to be the best one — it's just the

---

4   Merriam-Webster. (n.d.) Opportunity. In *Merriam-Websiter.com dictionary*. Retrieved October 1 2020, from https://www.merriam-webster.com/dictionary/opportunity

5   Eagleman, D. (2017, October). Understanding the neuroscience that fuels creative thinking can make you more innovative. [Post]. LinkedIn. https://www.linkedin.com/pulse/understanding-neuroscience-fuels-creative-thinking-can-david-eagleman/

one your brain arrived at fastest and without much difficulty. If you put your brain into a narrow and fixed mindset as you operate from a place of stress, you're sure to make it even more difficult to find solutions. Instead, by framing pain or weakness as an opportunity, you invite a more expansive growth mindset to allow solutions to present themselves that you may not have otherwise thought of. And adopting a growth mindset has far-reaching positive impacts on nearly every aspect of your life.

A growth mindset is one where you believe that you can influence things about yourself based on the effort you put into them, whereas a fixed mindset is one where you believe everything about yourself is set and that you have no real ability to change them. According to research done by psychologist Carol Dweck, who shared much of this research in her book *Mindset*, the impact of operating with a growth mindset is big. Not only do you learn more things at a faster rate when you operate with a growth mindset, you also are more motivated to put in effort, even when the thing you are working towards is quite substantial. And with a growth mindset, you're able to recognize that the journey is what matters — not just the outcome.

Says Dweck, "In the fixed mindset, everything is about the outcome. If you fail — or if you're not the best — it's all been wasted. The growth mindset allows people to value what they're doing regardless of the outcome. They're tackling problems, charting new courses, working on important issues. Maybe they haven't found the cure for cancer, but the search was deeply meaningful."[6]

So what do areas of opportunity and a growth mindset have to do with experiments you're going to be doing with your body? When you discover something about yourself that you want to try and impact through an experiment, and you choose to see it as an area of opportunity, you're more likely to:

- Learn from setbacks (and there will be setbacks — anyone telling you otherwise is trying to put one over on you)
- Stay focused without distraction (the world is full of distractions trying to steal your attention away from the thing you set out to do in the first place)
- Take ownership of the process (something you'll lean on frequently as you strike a balance between listening to experts in the field and trusting that you know what's best for you)

And in addition to all of this, there is much more you get from identifying areas of opportunity in your body. If your feet are hurting, the opportunity is obviously to figure out how to make your feet stop hurting. But your achy feet are also an opportunity to:

- Increase your knowledge about the feet and various

---

6 Dweck, C. (2007) *Mindset: The New Psychology of Success.* (Updated Edition) New York City, New York: Ballantine Books

things that influence how the bones and tissues in that area respond

- Become more attentive to your feet, and the rest of your body, as you implement a strategy to address the pain
- Improve your ability to be patient as you accept the reality of the time it takes to heal and improve
- Raise your body awareness as you learn more about what your body needs to feel and move its best

And so, simply by posing the question, "What's the opportunity?" a world of, well, opportunities opens up to you. However you decide to answer that question, your response will make your lantern burn brighter and you'll be able to see a direction worth heading. Whether it's to start doing something, to stop doing something, to switch something, to learn something… whether it's to tackle one of your signals directly, to tackle some other part of your health, your mind, your habits, or your lifestyle… the opportunity is the invitation. But is it an invitation to go it alone or to find someone to go with you? This brings us to the final question: *"who can help?"*

Who?

As a young adult, doctors would tell me each time I was in for an appointment, sick once again, that "This is just the way you are." They'd hand me yet another course of medication and shoo me out of their offices.

That's just the way I am? So 'just the way I am' is sick, exhausted, constantly dealing with infections, constantly taking antibiotics, experiencing muscle aches, stomach pains, and random signs of dis-ease?

This didn't make sense, and it certainly didn't jive with what I envisioned for myself. I knew it wasn't going to help my journey to become Unbreakable to have practitioners on the journey with me whose expectations of health, wellbeing, and feeling good were lower than my own. I don't blame those doctors. In fact, I thank them for teaching me that I need to be discerning about who I let join me on my journey.

Using discernment can be challenging at first, because you will often only know one path and one type of person to talk to regarding the area of opportunity you're facing. For example, if you only know about orthopedic surgeons, that's what you'll likely consider first. In some instances, that's the right first thing to consider, and in other instances, it might not be. And so, you'll need to explore as you consider who can help you, by learning about different types of experts and their specialties.

In addition, you'll need to cultivate your own set of values about body care and then seek out people who align with your values. And while you certainly could seek out people who align with your political values, that's not what I'm referring to here. Do you value taking a conservative approach to body care at first, or do you value hitting the thing you're dealing with hard with more invasive technologies? Do you value more traditional Western medicine or do you value Eastern philosophies of medicine? Do you value someone with good bedside manner or do you not value bedside manner at all as long as you get the treatment you need?

Cultivating and knowing your personal values in how you care for your body is a cornerstone of building your personal autonomy and it's an unavoidable part of the journey to become Unbreakable. It's an arena where other people have strong opinions that are rooted in their values, and as is often the case with opinions, folks like to give you theirs. But at the end of the day, it's *your* body. You get to decide what you do with it and how you take care of it.

After struggling with being 'just the way I was' for so many years, I reached a point where I knew who I didn't want on the journey with me but I didn't yet know who I did want. Who would have knowledge and expertise I'd like to receive? So, while I continued exploring to see if I could find anyone who might be able to help me, I got started with helping myself. And so, my answer to this final question in 'Three What's & A Who' —- 'who can help?' — was me.

My weekday evenings in those early years were spent looking things up online, going down rabbit holes on all manner of topics, and finding book after book to learn from that helped me select experiments to try. Over time, 'Who can help?' went from 'just me' to 'me and these folks who wrote blogs, shared stories, authored a book, or linked to an expert I'd never heard of but whose work sent me down the whole research cycle all over again.' Of course, not every blog, article, or book, was perfectly suited for me, but I took what was useful and left the rest.

Later, I found local practitioners I could work with directly, and 'Who can help?' became 'me and this practitioner.' As time has gone on, there have been other books, blogs, courses, and people who I've brought on the journey with me, but no matter what stage of the journey I've been at, answering the question 'Who can help?' has always included 'me'. And the answer to your 'Who can help?' question will always include you.

What a relief to know you're not on this journey alone! You may need to seek out some information, or find a practitioner, coach, teacher, or doctor to help you move forward because, of course, you're not expected to know everything. But in the end, you are on this journey with your body and nothing is ever entirely out of your hands.

Even in the case of a catastrophic accident, if you are alive, there is something you can do to help yourself move forward. It might be something as simple (yet profound) as learning to manage your thoughts at a time when all else seems to be out of control. It might be re-exploring your inner and outer environments to learn the changes they've been through since you last explored your body ecosystem. No matter what, there will always be a spot for you to join yourself on the journey to becoming Unbreakable.

The 'Three What's & A Who' questioning framework helps you set the stage for doing your experiment, which will come next. Before we dive into that, note that 'Three What's & A Who' also works on those stories and emotions you took note of when you were exploring and collecting data earlier.

I find using it on stories and emotions to be a lot like when you do a closet clean up — at first you're staring at a huge mess that feels like there is no good place to start. But then you begin to take things out one by one. You might have some nostalgic memories as you do so, and then you get to the business of organizing them into useful groups. Eventually, you can see clearly what can head to the trash bin, and with what remains you're able to figure out a reasonable way of reorganizing it.

Let me give you an example from the time when I was healing that ACL injury. There were days when the dominant worry in my mind was, "What if I can't do the activities I love anymore because this injury permanently alters how my body functions?"

This worry might seem over the top to anyone not in the middle of an injury — people recover from all kinds of far more serious events than this and go on to live wonderful and fulfilling lives. But that's the thing about stories and emotions: when left unchecked, they can really take hold and make things that are far-fetched seem not only real, but probable.

I used the questioning framework to unpack this story.

External signals that contributed to this worry was that first, I felt very far physically from where I needed to be to do the activities I loved. Second, lots of people experience an injury and *don't* get back to full capacity (note that my brain conveniently overlooked that lots of people *do* get back to full capacity).

The main internal signal that seemed to contribute to this worry was that, for most of my life, I was really good at catastrophizing. That is, my brain had learned to draw a fully detailed picture of the absolute worst possible scenario, but it was only able to draw a stick-figure picture of all the other scenarios that *weren't* that worst case scenario.

The opportunity, then, was to practice what I preach, to stick to the program of sending signals to my body, trusting that my body will respond, and believing in myself that I'll figure this out, one way or the other.

And finally, who can help was of course myself, but I also found a friend who helped me along the way as well, who you'll hear about in just a moment. Even just going through these questions helped me to feel more in control and capable, and then as I implemented experiments to try and influence this worry, my confidence as the one who is in control of what comes next grew.

Let's do a few more examples of body responses and the Three What's & A Who questioning framework to give you more practice in thinking about experiments for your body:

Example 1:

Body response: In Jamie's ongoing exploration of her inner and outer environments, she noticed a headache creeping in a few hours ago that is now going full bore between her temples.

Headaches can have very specific causes for some folks and seem to be quite nebulous for others. A pain-reliever can really help a headache in some cases, but you can't reverse that as easily and say that a lack of pain-relieving medication is the cause of the headache. (There is the case of when a person is detoxing from a drug that they can have horrific headaches because they don't have that drug in their system anymore. This is not what I'm referring to here.)

Here's Jamie's 'Three What's & A Who' to gain more context and identify possible experiments to do:

External: Didn't sleep as well last night, so perhaps that's it.

Internal: Too much coffee? Or perhaps, not enough coffee. Too little water today? I'm kind of stressed out and I do tend to clench my jaw more when stressed.

The opportunity: To check in with myself about my stress level, body care, and to see if I can figure out how to get rid of this headache and learn something about my body and its needs.

Who can help: Me, plus the people I find in my internet research who've done articles and videos about headaches.

Example 2:

Body response: Mark's back pain has been ongoing for months now, and not for lack of trying to resolve it.

This is a good example of how you can still make good use of your Explorer's Mindset, even if you've already tried a few things to influence your body's responses.

Here's Mark's '3 What's & A Who' to gain more context and identify possible experiments to do:

External: Bad office desk chair? Already bought a new chair to what seems like no avail. Bad mattress? Already switched the mattress, better, but not a complete resolution. High stress life lately? Haven't done much with this one yet.

Internal: Back muscles too weak? Tried a strength program already but maybe I could revisit this with a coach. Read an article about how pain can be about non-physical stuff, too. Not sure what this is about but I could get the book the article recommended. Something going on in my spine itself? Already talked to a doc and they said I've got some age-related degeneration that is to be expected, but to come back if my symptoms worsen.

The opportunity: To be patient as I keep trying to figure this out, to find a way to keep moving and living life even if my back doesn't change anytime soon, to appreciate the days when the pain is less disruptive, to find more experts who know about back pain and learn from them.

Who can help: Me and the experts I seek out to help me.

Example 3:

This one is an example of a story response: in Kirsten's exploration of her inner and outer environments, she collected some data about a worry she has. Her data was about how her body hurts but she keeps on pushing with her workouts, which to her doesn't seem like how it's supposed to be. Along with it was the worry that if she didn't keep pushing she'd be a failure.

Here's Kirsten's 'Three What's & A Who' to gain more context and identify possible experiments to do:

External: If I think back on my past, has anyone made me feel like I had to keep going even if I felt hurt? No, I can't remember anyone telling me that.

Internal: I remember being super dedicated as an athlete when I was a kid, which seemed to please my parents. It did feel good to get that praise and approval from Mom and Dad, and I liked being the best so maybe being super dedicated is something that's impacting me here? Is it possible to be dedicated but not be so stringent about my efforts? Not sure.

Thinking more in current times now, if I'm being honest I'm burning the candle at both ends because I'm so go-go-go in my efforts to do an awesome job at work, home, and in my fitness. I push to meet intense deadlines and I often feel like I'm barely even breathing as I push hard to get through my day. And because my day is so packed, I really have to hustle to fit my workout in and don't have any time for deviations. Is there a way to give my best efforts without having to feel so maxed out? That would be great but I don't really know how to do that.

The opportunity: To figure out if maybe there's another way to go about things that doesn't require me to keep it pinned to the point that I can't listen to my body's response of pain because it slows me down, to learn something about myself and why I do the things I do.

Who can help: Me, and I think I'll bring this book on mindfulness and busy-ness that a friend recommended to me on board to help me get started.

CHAPTER 7:

Testing, Testing, 1, 2, 3...

Now that you've prepped yourself to do an experiment, it's time to go over the process of experimenting. Do you recall the scientific method from your grade school biology class? Don't worry if not, I've drawn it out on the next page.

The scientific method is a structured way of doing experiments and seeing what the results are. Being able to do a good experiment is invaluable for really learning what your body responds best to. It might be tempting to just wing it, but this isn't a pot of stew where you just throw in a bit of this and a handful of that and call it good. This is about cultivating a level of expertise in taking care of your body ecosystem that no one other than you could ever have about yourself.

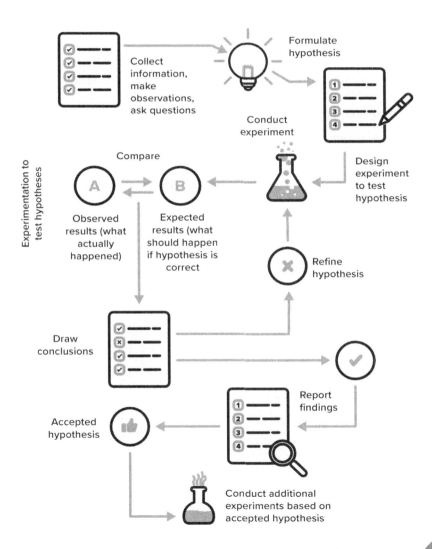

Collect information, make observations, ask questions

Formulate hypothesis

Design experiment to test hypothesis

Conduct experiment

Compare

Experimentation to test hypotheses

A — Observed results (what actually happened)

B — Expected results (what should happen if hypothesis is correct

Refine hypothesis

Draw conclusions

Report findings

Accepted hypothesis

Conduct additional experiments based on accepted hypothesis

Experiments for your body can run the gamut:

- Starting a workout program
- Making a change to your bedtime routine
- Choosing a new way of eating
- Beginning a meditation practice
- Switching out your shoes or your desk chair
- Setting up physical therapy appointments, and so on.

Everything you do with the goal of helping yourself is an experiment. Even the actions you take that don't get you the response you desire are a useful experiment because they give you more knowledge about your body and how it responds to a particular signal. And if you're still hoping for some magical option that will ensure you never choose an experiment that goes awry, consider this: the only way you will learn to manage your stressors is by struggling with your stressors.

The only way you'll learn which foods make you feel the way you want to feel is by realizing certain foods don't make you feel that way and tinkering with your meals. The only way you'll improve at something is by doing that something. As my friend Kathryn Dixon, founder of Clarity Coaching Institute, once put it, "How will you learn how to handle something new if you never let yourself handle something new?" Ain't that the truth.

To do your first experiment, take a look at the list of things you noted when you answered the first two What questions about external and internal signals. Which one stands out as the first thing you'd like to tackle? By selecting a signal to try and influence or change, you're setting your hypothesis.

Hypotheses are just educated guesses that are testable. In formal scientific experiments, a hypothesis is usually written as an 'if this, then that' statement, as in "if I change my shoes, switching out these dress shoes for a sneaker, then my feet will feel better." When you choose a signal to experiment with, what you're saying is that you think you'll get the response you desire if you alter this particular signal in some way.

Once you've chosen your signal and thus set your hypothesis, it's time to set the parameters for the experiment. (Sidenote: this whole process becomes much more automatic once you have done it a few times. We're just going through the intricate specifics now so you learn the process in full.) Parameters for an experiment are important because they keep things from getting messy.

You already know that it's often a web of signals which influences the kind of response your body is making. And so, when doing an experiment to see if you can learn something about what makes your body respond in a different way, it pays to keep as many variables of the experiment as steady as you can.

For example:

- How often in a given day or week will you do/not do the thing you're experimenting with?

- How strenuously will you do the thing?
- Will you stop doing anything else while you do this experiment?
- Where in your day will you place your experiment each day that you do it?
- What other aspects of life do you need to account for in your experiment?
- What piece of data will tell you that you can stop running the experiment now and evaluate its outcome?

Parameters help you set the structure for your experiment. They also help you know when you've collected enough data from the experiment to determine if it worked the way you'd hoped. At some point, you need to know 'this worked well and I have enough data to draw a conclusion now' or 'this didn't work out as I'd hoped and it's time to try something else.'

As an example, when I was rehabbing my ACL, I decided to do some work with a physical therapist friend of mine. She was uniquely talented in providing care that integrated nervous system regulation and a level of calm restoration to the body that I just didn't find with other practitioners and so my 'Who can help' answer included her for a period of time.

My hypothesis was that my friend's expertise and talent would aid the rehab work I was already doing, and the outcome of the experiment would be that I'd feel better and I'd make more progress in my healing journey. I tested the hypothesis by going for weekly visits, and indeed I felt things improving for me. My parameter for deciding when to stop this experiment was when it had either worked so well that there isn't much difference between my regular training and what we're doing in the sessions, or until four weeks had passed if no change was experienced.

I hit the four-week mark and decided to keep going because I was absolutely experiencing change. Eventually, we had reduced the pain, built up a lot of capacity, and my training now looked more like strength and conditioning than it did rehab. We had hit the parameter I'd set and so, it was time to finish the sessions. This experiment was complete and I was pleased with the outcome.

Had we hit the four-week parameter I'd set and I'd not experienced change, I'd have moved on to the next experiment on my list, feeling glad to know that I didn't have to keep doing something that wasn't working for me. Parameters are how you make decisions like knowing when to call an experiment 'complete'.

This brings us to the next steps in your experimentation process — actually doing the experiment and collecting the results. Run your experiment for however long you decided was 'long enough' to see if it gave you the response you were after. And as you do, observe and collect data. How is the area of opportunity you're experimenting on feeling? Better? Same? Worse? Have there been any other noticeable changes, to your body, your mood, your mind, your energy, or anything else? How are *you* feeling? Are you having fun?

(Oh, you didn't realize that experimenting could actually be fun? It can be!)

As you run the experiment, take stock of what's happening by continuing to collect data about things that are changing. It can be as simple as noticing that your hip or back feels one percent better today than yesterday or it can be more particular, perhaps you try a particular motion like raising your leg up in the air each week and evaluate the degree to which the range of motion increased from the previous week. At the end of your experiment, you'll compare your actual results to your expected results.

And whichever way the experiment goes, you've got options. Either your hypothesis hit the bullseye you were aiming for, or it didn't. Whichever way it went, you can draw some conclusions. If you proved your hypothesis, then the next steps are to either keep doing the action or stop the action if it's no longer necessary.

If the action you took in your experiment is one of those "this is a good practice to keep up in my life" things, then adopt it as part of your life and carry on. Things like my daily movement series and heading out into nature regularly are that for me. Or if the action you took in your experiment was more in the realm of "this helps me heal, but once I'm healed, it's not necessary anymore", then you'll stop doing it after you've healed. Like wearing a cast on a broken arm, these are practices that are helpful for healing but not necessary, or even ideal, after healing has occurred. They serve you as needed and then are left behind as you progress forward on your journey.

Shoot, It Didn't Work The Way I'd Hoped

Let's talk now about what to do when the experiment doesn't give you the results you were aiming for — either it hits the target but is way off the bullseye, or it's nowhere near the target at all. First, even if it didn't create the results you hoped for, it still 'worked,' in that you got helpful information out of the experiment. You see, if changing your shoes made no difference in your foot pain, and you met the parameters for how long you were going to do the experiment before deciding if it achieved the outcome you intended, then you've narrowed down the potential signals contributing to your foot pain by one. It appears that it's not your shoes, at least not in this instance. Good to know. Now you can turn your attention to the next signal you identified as a possible contributor to your foot pain when you did the Three What's & A Who questions.

And if you've already gone through all the signals you identified in Three What's & A Who, then it's time to do some more exploring to learn more about the body response you're experiencing and what else could influence it in the way you desire. Being an explorer means being inquisitive about what you know you don't know yet, and being open to curiosity about all the things you don't even know that you don't know yet.

What about trying a bunch of experiments at once to try and multiply your success? There is a time and place for 'stacking' of experiments where you do a few or several things at once, to be sure. In the case of my ruptured ACL, I already knew how lots of different signals worked for me from past education and experimentation, so I could stack them straight away and feel fairly confident in the outcome I'd get from doing so.

As you learn which signals make a particular response for you, you'll develop a better sense of how to pair two or more signals together and get a combination that works beautifully to help you maintain your Unbreakable body. In addition, you'll develop a hierarchy of the various signals, with the most impactful ones at the top of the list. This makes it easier to beeline for those signals the next time you find yourself needing to take action to address an undesirable response.

However, stacking is not the same as what I call 'kitchen sinking it'. A thought might be simmering in your mind at this point: "If experimenting with one signal is good, experimenting with *all* the signals at once must be better!" When you're experiencing pain, it can be tempting to throw everything and the kitchen sink at this response you wish to rid yourself of. If your back is hurting, you might think that if you switch your office chair, start doing stretches, book in weekly massages, start holding your body in 'better posture' positions, and take ibuprofen all at the same time, that you'll get results faster than if you experimented with just one signal at a time.

This is the epitome of 'kitchen sinking' it — throwing as many things as you can at a problem and simply by the law of probability, you're bound to have chosen at least one that 'works' to get rid of the pain you're dealing with.

If you're confident in what kinds of responses these signals cultivate in your body, then by all means, have at it. But if you've not experimented with the signals before and thus don't have a history of knowing how they work for you, an issue may arise. Let's say you 'kitchen sink' it and your back starts to feel better. Hooray! You stop the ibuprofen, massage, and stretches, and you go on about your life.

But then the pain returns. Oh no! Now you've got a whole new set of questions to answer. Which signal or signals was making the biggest impact for you? Which ones should you start with on this second foray into back pain? If you've got this new chair, but the pain is back again, was the chair even the issue in the first place?

Put another way, if your objective is to get responses you prefer by making the biggest, widest spray of effort possible, with signals you know work for you, 'kitchen sink' it. But if your objective is to get responses you prefer *and* to learn how particular signals work for you, be mindful of doing so many things at once that you can't tell what's working for you.

CHAPTER 8:

Curating Results To Craft Your Personal Plan For Success

By collecting a wealth of data about your body ecosystem, and accumulating information about how your body responds to various experiments, you're not only able to come up with a unique and customized protocol for caring for your Unbreakable body, you start tapping into the benefits of having that deep-seated wisdom about your body, and you automatically improve your skill set around exploring and experimenting.

You're able to notice something like not getting great sleep the last few days, and knowing what to watch out for in your body responses today. Because you've got history with knowing how your body responds, you might know that the sleep issue tends to make you feel more stiff and achy, and so if you then do feel more stiff and achy during your day, you don't have to worry about it. "Yep, to be expected since I haven't been sleeping well, it will resolve on its own once I get a great night of sleep or two."

With this wisdom you also can make adjustments on the fly because you know the ways in which your body has responded to similar signal shifts in the past. This is one reason why aches and injuries and 'stuff you don't like' are such a gift: in your efforts to heal, tend to, and eliminate the stuff you don't like, you learn so much about how your body responds.

"Well, I haven't slept great so instead of the normal workout I was going to do today, I'll switch it for the Yoga & Chill class they have at the studio tonight." If you already know that the Yoga & Chill class helps you get a better night's sleep and it makes you feel like you still moved your body, even if you didn't do the workout you planned, then it's a no-brainer to shift gears and head to class.

In addition, when you notice a body response that you really don't like, you're able to run through your list of signals and assess if you've been doing everything that you know usually makes your body respond in the manner you'd prefer.

For instance, if you've noticed that your feet are achy and tired lately, you can run through your list of signals you know usually help your feet feel great. Have I been wearing different shoes? Have I been doing the foot exercises I learned in my workout program? Have I been on my feet more than usual?

With these curated protocols of signals that worked for you in the past, you can re-examine them and catch something that you might have been doing before but stopped doing, or which signals need the dial turned up.

As you curate the information you're getting out of your exploration and experiments, you're also able to more quickly hypothesize about what your body might need from you when you notice a body response that you'd like to do something about. And, you become able to do it so quickly that it just feels intuitive — like the elderly Grandma making her famous spaghetti sauce just *knows* whether it needs more garlic or basil.

This Seems Like It's Going To Take A Long Time... Is There A Faster Route?

When you want something — and wanting relief from the aches and pains is a worthy 'something' to want — you probably would prefer to get it sooner rather than later. I get it. And it's understandable to feel your frustration rise as you just want to solve the problem *now*. As someone who once held a seat on the board of the Society Of Impatient People, I know all about that frustration.

Experiments are a process of funneling. You're trying to funnel down to the most valuable actions that create the responses you desire in your body. The more experiments you do, the more you are funneling your actions, and the closer you are getting to the thing that will produce the outcome you desire.

And if you're thinking, "But I want the fastest route to fixing my problem, er, area of opportunity," believe me when I say that this *is* the fastest route. There are no shortcuts to becoming an expert in anything, including becoming an expert in You. In her book, *Sacred Success*, Barbara Stanny writes, "Impatience — like perfectionism — is fear based."[7]

You get impatient when you want something faster than the speed it's going at. You get impatient when you want to grip tightly to control in the hopes that if you grip hard enough, you'll get what you want. You get impatient when reality doesn't match your expectations.

But rather than hate your impatience, apply some curious compassion to it and I think you'll see that impatience is simply desire that's in a hurry to get somewhere.

And in case all this talk of experimenting narrowed your focus a bit from the real opportunity at hand, allow me to remind you. You are the explorer of your body. No one has

7   Stanny. B (2014) *Sacred Success: A Course In Financial Miracles*. Dallas, Texas: BenBella Books

ever been here before. It's your job to figure this place out, to make it hospitable for you. The opportunity is to get relief from your aches and pains to get strong for the life you want, *and* to learn about yourself and what it takes to take care of this body you're living in.

As the explorer of your body, go explore! Become familiar with the environments, both inner and outer, in which you live. With each experiment, you learn something, you become wiser, more capable, and you take another stop on your journey to becoming Unbreakable. Yes, it can feel frustrating to have the journey take longer than you'd wish. Yes, it can feel scary to try something and find that it doesn't create the outcome you were hoping for when it seemed to work fine for someone else. Yes, it can feel like a burden you didn't ask for.

But what's the alternative? Really think about it for a moment: what's the alternative to being an explorer of your body and performing experiments to figure out how to make life in your body as hospitable for you as possible? To be a passenger on the ride. To have life happen to you without happening back at it. To let go of the leadership role that is inherent to you as the caretaker of your body. A hearty 'no thanks' to that.

Now that you know it's not too late for you, and you've got a method for exploring, experimenting, and curating, it's time to tackle that whole 'it's too complicated for you' myth. In part three of this book, it's time to shift from awareness to action and look into those impactful conversations you're having every day with your body that influence how you feel, how you heal, how you move, and what you can do.

Before we close the chapter, let's recap how we got to where we are. You know now that bodies always respond to the signals they receive by way of the nervous system, and so tending to both the system and the signals is how you can make a big impact in your body responses. To do so, you'll need to start exploring and collecting data about the responses you're noticing in both your inner and outer environments. You'll even take stock of those emotion-driven stories, beliefs, worries, and fears you have about your body and its parts, experiences, and areas of opportunity.

Once you select a piece of data you'd like to influence, you'll seek out context for the data and organize your ideas around what signals might be contributing to that response. You'll get your mind focused towards growth, you'll get clear on the opportunity that lies before you, and you'll consider who might be useful to help you on this part of the journey.

You'll then set your experiment up to send the signals you think will influence the response you're experimenting on in a favorable way. Upon running your experiment to completion, you'll find out if the hypothesis you were testing with your experiment was correct. If it was, you get to decide now if that signal is one that you'll want to keep communicating to your body because it's something that's ideal for the long-term, or if the signal can be stopped now because you've healed the part of your body that was dealing with the response you didn't prefer. And if your hypothesis wasn't correct and you've still got a body response you don't prefer, it's time to move on to the next signal you identified in your list, set up a new experiment and note the results.

Remember to keep track of all of it in your Unbreakable Field Journal (whether a real notebook or just a mental note in your mind) as you become the expert of this amazing body ecosystem you're living in. Let's set off now for conversations with your body. We're going to begin with the conversation of pain (I know, how fun!).

Believe it or not, learning about pain can actually make you more effective and efficient in the other conversations you're having with your body. Then we'll get into the conversation about building your body, physically, and finally, building that non-physical stuff that really bolsters you as the Unbreakable human you are.

PART THREE:

Communication With Your Body

CHAPTER 9:

The Conversation You're In With Your Body

Think about the last time you communicated with another person. What were you doing in communicating with them? You were trying to pass information to them to get them to know or do something — understand you, let them know you understand them, teach them, express interest in them, etc. Even non-verbal communication comes with the same end-goal, an exchange of information. And communication is not relegated to something that is done between two humans or a human and their pet.

You and your body, including your nerves, bones, tissues, organs, even your thoughts, are communicating every day. This isn't just "say nice things to yourself" stuff though, although kind self-talk does support you better than negative self-talk. The type of communication you'll mostly be doing with your body is that of actions, not words. The signals you're sending to your body are a form of communication, as is how your body responds. Whether you're intentional about the signals you send to your body or not, it's all a form of communication.

It's through this communication by way of signals, that information is passed to your body, and with that information your body responds. The accumulation of these responses is how you create adaptations and it's these adaptations that turn you into the Unbreakable vision you have for yourself.

But where to begin? What communication can you send that will move you closer to your vision of becoming Unbreakable? We can't cover every possible communication between you and your body in just one book, but we'll focus on the most impactful conversations you're having every day that influence how you feel, how you heal, how you move, and what you can do. And through these conversations you'll be able to influence a wide variety of responses your body is experiencing.

To do so, we must begin at the nervous system. All of the

communication you'll have with your body will flow by way of your nervous system. It's almost a disservice to name a few of the things your nervous system does because these are just a drop in the highly complex bucket of actions your nervous system delivers every day.

Nonetheless, here are a few:

- Breathing
- Thinking
- Experiencing emotions
- Sensing the temperature of the room you're sitting in
- Controlling your movement
- Balance and coordination
- Changing the tonicity or 'tightness' in a muscle
- Increasing and decreasing your heart rate
- Vision changes
- Creating painful sensations.

In short, your nervous system is how you sense your surroundings and respond accordingly. All communication you send to your body to help it become Unbreakable will run through the nervous system, and every response you experience comes by way of the nervous system. So let's go through a simple overview of the nervous system, so that you've got your bearings before we head off into the particulars of the most impactful conversations you're having with your body.

Meet Your Nervous System

This is where we start laying the groundwork for you to make changes to how you feel and move in your body. We're going to get into a bit of science, but remember: nothing is 'too complicated' for you. While this might seem detailed, you don't have to memorize it to be able to move forward. This information is simply here to help you make the necessary changes later on to become Unbreakable.

Your nervous system is made up of your brain, spinal cord, and nerves, and it's through these components of your nervous system that information is received, synthesized, and responded to. Your nervous system participates in literally everything you do. Your brain and spinal cord are called your central nervous system, or CNS.

The ganglia (which are groups of neuron cell bodies) and nerves that branch out from your spinal cord, extending out to muscles and organs, are called your peripheral nervous system. Your central nervous system plays a primary role in receiving information from various areas of the body and then coordinating this activity to produce the body's responses.

Your peripheral nervous system's primary role is to connect the central nervous system to the organs, limbs, and skin. These nerves extend from the central nervous system to the outermost areas of the body. From this point, there are many branches of the nervous system, so here's a picture to refer back to.

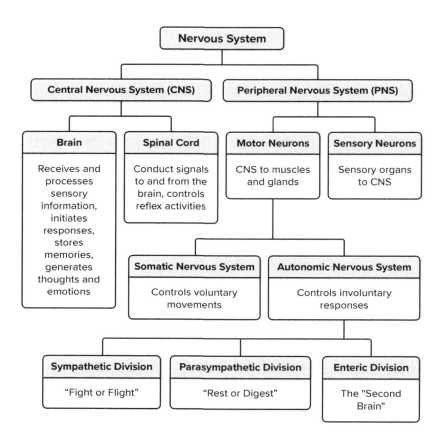

The peripheral nervous system is divided into two divisions: the afferent (sensory) division and an efferent (motor) division.

The afferent or sensory division transmits impulses from peripheral organs to the CNS. The efferent or motor division transmits impulses from the CNS out to the peripheral organs to cause an effect or action.[8] Finally, the efferent or motor division is again subdivided into the somatic system, which controls all voluntary muscle actions and muscle reflexes in your body, and the autonomic system, which regulates involuntary bodily functions like heart rate, digestion, and body temperature regulation.

Both of these branches are constantly sending information to your central nervous system via afferent nerves and receiving information back via efferent nerves.

Next, within your autonomic nervous system there are three branches (I know, stay with me):

1) the sympathetic nervous system, commonly known as the 'fight or flight' system
2) the parasympathetic nervous system, also called the 'rest and digest' system, and
3) the enteric nervous system, which you've probably heard referred to as 'the second brain' (it resides in your gastrointestinal tract and operates independently of the central nervous system, although the two do communicate with and influence each other).

You have probably heard that you shift into the 'fight or flight' system when a stressful event occurs, and you shift into 'rest and digest' when the stressful event has passed.

---

8 SEER Training Modules, Organization Of The Nervous System. U. S. National Institutes of Health, National Cancer Institute. 1 Oct 2021 Retrieved from https://www.training.seer.cancer.gov/anatomy/nervous/organization/

Earlier in human history the stressful event was usually an intense but short-lived event: narrowly escaping a grizzly bear charging at you. But these days, while you might still experience intense events (though not very likely to involve grizzly bears) you're more likely to experience low-level but chronic stressors: financial worries, the ongoing stress of a job you hate and so on.

Regardless of the size of the threat, and regardless of whether it's real or imagined, when you face something you perceive as threatening, your nervous system responds accordingly. There are several common physiological changes that occur when you ramp up into the sympathetic nervous system, including the release of hormones like adrenaline and cortisol, increased muscle tension, shallower and faster breathing, and the de-prioritization of functions not critical to survival. In addition, you're likely to change how you move and position yourself to make you more ready to respond, including extending your spine and raising up on the balls of your feet.

Just think of how you move your body if someone surprises you or startles you. Your spine tightens up and moves into an extended position, and even if you're seated, you likely jump a little bit as you startle. You can't jump from your heels, so even if seated, your weight will shift towards your toes. Once the threat has passed, it's time to restore calm in your body so you can do other important things that your body needs to do to survive and thrive. Your body positioning will move away from that extended spine position, you'll relax back into the heels of your feet, and your parasympathetic system will slow down your heart rate, relax your muscles, and start clearing excess adrenaline from your body. This helps you to feel calm, relaxed, restful, and present, amongst other good-feeling characteristics.

The harmonious oscillation between these two branches of the autonomic nervous system is known as self-regulation, whereas being 'stuck' in one branch of the autonomic nervous system is known as dysregulation. When you can self-regulate, your body will adjust and adapt to whatever conditions it is facing so that it can maintain a stable and consistent internal environment. This is known as homeostasis.

For example, if you go out walking on the hottest summer day, your body will engage in various mechanisms to cool your body temperature, including sweating and increasing the circulation of the blood to the surface of the body to allow for the dissipation of heat through the skin. These changes occur because the part of your brain monitoring body temperature, your hypothalamus, sensed your body temperature rising and set off processes to lower it.

When in a state of dysregulation, your nervous system responds to signals in a disproportionate manner, either as an underreaction or an overreaction to the situation at hand. To keep with the thermoregulation example, a dysregulated system might struggle to keep the hands and feet warm in cooler temperatures, or might create excessive body heat in a room others would call 'room temperature'.

But it's not just temperature that is being affected by dysregulation of the nervous system. Because your nervous system is a part of every aspect of your experience living in your body, symptoms can take many, many different forms. They include:

- Being hypervigilant and having extreme startle reactions
- Having trouble sleeping
- Feeling anxious or stressed out
- Experiencing exhaustion
- Being unable to focus for extended periods of time.

Symptoms can also manifest as physical changes like joint issues, muscle strains and pulls, tendonitis, chronic pain, digestion issues, vision issues, high blood pressure, pelvic floor issues, headaches, low heart rate variability, and it can even impact your emotions and mood.

Dr. James Anderson is a physical therapist who takes a neurocentric approach (meaning he works with the nervous system as a primary focus of attention) to address and resolve issues with the body. When I was visiting with him for my own body care needs, we got to talking about the nervous system and with his permission, I'm sharing parts of our conversation with you.

Regarding the nervous system and dysregulation, Dr. Anderson had this to say:

"When your nervous system is dysregulated, your system perceives a threat as a greater threat than it is. We see hypervigilance and hypersensitivity as symptoms of a hyper response to some signal. It's too much to manage."

And so, when it comes to building a body you love to live in, it's not just about sending signals so that you can get responses, you also want to ensure that the system that is processing those signals, ie, your nervous system, is able to manage the signals appropriately and respond appropriately. Your nervous system is more capable of doing so when it is able to oscillate between the sympathetic and parasympathetic branches of your nervous system.

Unfortunately, it's common to find yourself chronically stuck, ramped up in the sympathetic nervous system. It's not just momentous situations like "there is a grizzly bear in my kitchen" or "the boss has requested a gulp-inducing meeting with me" that ramp up your sympathetic nervous system. It can also ramp up based on any stressor that takes you away from homeostasis — from the barrage of emails, social media, news, and all of the other things you're 'supposed' to keep up with in life, and even things as seemingly unavoidable as how you take each of the 17,000+ breaths you take each day, or what sort of posture you assume with your body. Yes, even breathing and posture can have an impact on how your nervous system oscillates between the two branches of the autonomic nervous system.

Remember I mentioned earlier that you've got bundles of afferent nerves that are constantly sending information to the brain and spinal cord, and bundles of efferent nerves that are sending information from the brain and spinal cord to the rest of the body? Inside your ribcage running down either side of your spinal cord are big bundles of nerves called the sympathetic ganglia that are made up of these afferent and efferent nerves. Dr. Anderson describes the shape of the sympathetic ganglia as "a dangling bundle of Christmas lights. The lightbulbs in this case are bunches of nerves."

He went on to explain:

"These bunches of nerves can be compressed, and when compressed they will activate more of a sympathetic nervous system response. They can also be decompressed to deactivate the sympathetic nervous system response and to allow the nervous system to shift into the parasympathetic nervous system response. These bundles of nerves act like sensors for how the body needs to react to what's coming next."

So when you face a grizzly bear or the tax man and you innately alter your body position to raise up on your toes and extend your spine, you compress the bundles of nerves that make up the sympathetic ganglia, which ramps up your sympathetic nervous system.

The body position, in addition to making the structures

of your body more ready to fight or to flee, also tells your nervous system to trigger that sympathetic nervous system response of flooding you with adrenaline, releasing cortisol, and making your internal environment ready for fighting or fleeing as well.

Ironically, this compression also happens when you try to 'stand up straight' — pulling your shoulders back and thrusting your chest out in order to have 'good posture'. Despite there being no threat present and without intending for it to be the case, your 'good' posture creates an internal environment that is stuck more in a sympathetic nervous system response. But your nervous system doesn't know that — it's just responding to the signals it receives.

Breathing also can influence how the sympathetic ganglia are compressed. Due to their position, when your lungs expand as you inhale, they become compressed. Ideally, they become decompressed when you exhale, however, it's very common to have developed a mode of respiration that never fully decompresses the sympathetic ganglia. And so even something as simple as a breath can influence if you stay in the sympathetic nervous system, or whether you relax into the parasympathetic nervous system, all of which can influence how your nervous system overall responds to other signals you're sending to it. We'll talk more about optimal respiration and how to achieve it in a later chapter, but now that we've done a brief overview of your nervous system, we can add the next dimension to the Signal/Response Principle.

You know now that your body is always responding to the signals that it receives. And, you've learned about how regulated or dysregulated your nervous system is will play a role in how those signals and responses get processed. If you think of the regulation of the nervous system as a range that you can move along, with regulation more in the middle and dysregulation more on the ends, how your nervous system responds to the signals it receives is likely to be a bit different depending on where you're at in that range of regulation.

So, taking care of your body ecosystem means learning about three things — the signals you're sending, the responses you're receiving, and where you're at on the range of regulation (and a bonus fourth thing: learning what helps you move towards regulation if you find you are experiencing dysregulation).

Knowing that you can influence both the signals you send and the nervous system that you'll send them through is an incredible relief. I say relief because if you're not enjoying the responses you're experiencing, you can send new signals. And if you're sending signals and not liking the responses you're getting, not only do you have the opportunity to try other signals, you also have the opportunity to learn about your nervous system's regulation and try some signals to influence it to move in a direction you'd prefer as well.

In addition, if you know you're dealing with aspects of life right now that are making it so you're living more in that sympathetic driven stress response (it happens, life's a doozie sometimes), you can give yourself grace by knowing that your body is doing the best it can and currently, under these conditions, the response it's giving you is the best it can do.

Because truly, your body is never trying to hurt you. It's always trying to help you, and boy, that's a soothing perspective to take as opposed to hating your body for not doing what you want it to do. I know it might seem nonsensical that pain you feel is actually your body trying to be helpful, but it will make much more sense as we head into the next chapter, which all about pain.

We're going to start with the conversation of pain because understanding that clarifies all of the other conversations you and your body can have.

CHAPTER 10:

What Is Pain?

Pain isn't new. Since the dawn of human history, pain has been part of the human experience. There were those who had the misfortune to get munched on by a bear or lion while they were out hunting for their tribe. There were those who experienced the pain of starvation during a particularly harsh season. Some were shot in battle, others were bucked off their horse, and of course someone walked into poison ivy for the first time and dealt with the consequences.

There was also seemingly unexplainable pain in ancient history — pain that seemed to come out of nowhere and didn't have an easily identifiable cause. And while we don't know if ancient civilizations complained around the proverbial water cooler about their low back pain, we do know that some ancient humans believed that pain that showed up for no identifiable reason was a curse from the gods, from God with a capital G, from spirits, or from supernatural energies. Maybe there is some supernatural energy out there that just waits for you to turn 40 and then delivers a sack of aches and pains to you, and like the search for Bigfoot, we just haven't found the hard evidence yet. Doubtful, but you can believe it if you want to.

Now of course, if pain isn't new then neither is the act of trying to get rid of it. You, me, and countless humans that came before us have all had pain we wanted gone. If you had pain in ancient history, you might have seen a shaman or medicine woman, you might have done some bloodletting, you may have eaten certain plants, had your bones set, or said some incantations to your god of choice in the hopes of ridding yourself of the pain.

If you were alive in the 1800s, there was a good chance that if your pain was to be remedied with surgery, you went under the knife without anesthetic, and in an ironic twist you got to experience a level of pain that is almost unimaginable in order to resolve your original pain. Novelist Frances Bernay gave a good idea of what that kind of pain feels like, when she wrote to her sister about her experience of having a mastectomy without anesthesia. "I began a scream that lasted intermittently during the whole time of the incident — and I almost marvel that it rings not in my ears still! So excruciating was the agony." A knife to the chest will do that to a person.

Even neck pain — ever common in modern times — dates back to at least 1600 BCE, where a diagnostic test and treatment for a vertebral sprain in the neck is mentioned on the Edwin Smith Papyrus, which is the oldest known treatise on trauma. (The treatment for the vertebral sprain, as stated on the papyrus, was to "bind it in fresh meat on the first day.")

And just as humans have been exploring ways of treating pain since the dawn of time, so too have humans been debating where pain originates from. This is a worthy thing to consider if you believe that if you can figure out where it comes from, you'll be able to figure out how to stop it. But there's a small glitch when you look at pain as having a singular source — more on that in a moment. For Aristotle, pain was an emotion. For Descartes, pain was a disturbance that passed along the nerve fibers to the brain in a very mechanical sense. And by the mid-nineteenth century, pain and disease were predominantly viewed as solely biological events that had exclusively biomedical solutions.

What that meant was that if you had pain, the belief was that there was either some damage or dysfunction in your physiology or in your biochemistry, or your symptoms were being caused by the pathology of whatever disease you contracted. And in this biomedical model, the solution was to be found by examining and treating solely the biological condition.

This biomedical model considered pain to be a sensation that arises from some sort of pathology or damage to the tissues, and that the pain should be relative to the amount of tissue damage (that is, more damage should equal more pain and more pain should mean more damage to the tissue). This model does work in some instances, but it also leaves a lot of significant gaps.

For example, the biomedical model has a very hard time explaining phantom limb pain in individuals who have had an amputation. Or, imagine that you feel pain in your knee and you've had it for long enough and it hurts bad enough that you go see a doctor. You didn't know going in that the doctor is going to examine your knee through the lens of the biomedical model of pain. So, the doctor examines you and determines that there is no pathogen, tumor, or disease that has caused your knee pain. They also determine that there is no damage to your tissues that is causing your pain. They check out your body's biochemistry and can't find anything causing your pain.

"We can't find anything wrong", the doctor says as he completes his examination. "Come back if it gets worse." You're left with knee pain that feels very real to you, but the source of which is a mystery to this medical professional. And then what? Clearly, the biomedical approach to pain can leave a lot to be desired.

It was George L. Engel who, in 1977, introduced what is now known as the 'biopsychosocial model' (BPS model, for short) which suggests that disease and pain (and health and wellbeing) depend upon a range of things including biological, psychological and social factors, hence the name bio-psycho-social. Engel took what was formerly a single-focus approach (biological factors only) to disease, pain, and health, and added several more dimensions to it with his BPS model.

He suggested that to understand and treat disease and pain, one must look at much more than just physical factors like tissue damage, because the experience of pain is about more than just tissue damage. He suggested that the experience of pain can be influenced by a person's beliefs, thoughts, emotions and coping strategies, as well as things like psychological distress or fear they may be experiencing. He also noted that you must also look at the social and environmental factors the person is dealing with, like work issues, family circumstances, relationship with a partner, and living situation, as all of these things could be contributing to the sensation of pain, too.

The BPS model suggests that pain emerges as part of an experience that is unique to you and is highly influenced by broader issues embedded in the interactions among the biological, psychological, and social components which you're experiencing at this time.

There are many definitions and descriptions of pain that have been given over time, but I think this one in particular evokes a mental picture of how seemingly separate things can come together to form something else, as we see in the BPS model:

> "Pain is a complex constellation of unpleasant sensory, emotional and cognitive experiences provoked by real or perceived tissue damage and manifested by certain autonomic, psychological, and behavioral reactions."[9]

With a view through the BPS lens, you still treat your tissues, organs, and systems of your body, if and when they need treating, *and* you consider tending to other factors like a your stress level, your worries, your beliefs, if you're sleeping well, and other factors that seem at first glance to have nothing to do with a tissue injury. Tend to the entire ecosystem, and the individual components tend to improve.

It's worth mentioning that if you slipped with the kitchen knife while chopping onions and chopped into your finger, it probably hurts because you chopped your finger — not because you had a stressful day at work. At that acute moment, other factors in your life probably aren't influencing your pain levels in the same way that the bleeding gash in your finger is. But how long it hurts after the fact, and how long it takes to heal, is influenced by the information coming to your brain and how your brain is processing it in the wider context of your life.

---

9   1Fishman, Ballantyne, and Rathmell (2010) Bonica's Management of Pain. 3rd ed. Philadelphia, Pennsylvania: Lippincott Williams and Wilkins

Overflowing Cups

Pain tells you that something is going on and your attention is needed. It can help you become aware of changes you might want to make. And while pain can certainly feel annoying, frustrating, and quite uncomfortable, if you didn't ever feel pain, that would be a much greater problem.

If you touch a hot stove, you feel a painful sensation and before you even think to do it, you're pulling your hand away from the heat. That's your somatic nervous system at work responding reflexively to the hot temperature on your skin. Now imagine if you didn't sense anything while your hand was on the hot stove. Your skin tissue would burn and you'd develop a wound. If you kept doing this over and over again because you didn't recognize when you were burning your skin, you'd be rolling the dice that one of those wounds would become infected, which could become life-threatening. And so, having your nervous system alert you to possible threats is vital. But not all perceived threats are as straightforward as 'hot thing hurts, pull hand away'.

Today, pain is viewed as an *opinion* of the brain because the brain thinks you may be in danger, and so it does something to protect you from the perceived threat. It is an outcome of a multitude of bits of information that have made their way to your brain, where your brain has processed them, synthesized them, and responded to them in a manner it deems appropriate.

As that information is being processed, your brain is asking, "How much of a threat is this?" If your brain decides the information indicates enough of a threat that it should protect you, it creates the sensation of pain — which you might feel in your low back area, your knee, your neck, your shoulder, or anywhere else in your body. But the sticky point here is your brain responding 'in a manner it deems appropriate'.

The notion of what's appropriate will vary from person to person, generation to generation, and culture to culture. What I deem appropriate may not be what you deem appropriate. Your brain, my brain, and all the brains out there are deciding each day 'what's appropriate' with regard to how they will respond to the signals they receive.

And as you now know, how your nervous system is operating will influence how the system responds to the signal it receives, and the way your nervous system responds will be different to how somebody else's nervous system responds. Many things can contribute to your brain forming the opinion that creating a painful sensation is appropriate, and those 'many things' do not have to include physical damage to tissues. Yes, really — you can feel a painful sensation that has no tissue-specific cause. And even more interestingly, you can have tissue-specific issues, like disc degeneration and protrusion, meniscus abnormalities, muscle tears, and similar such issues throughout your body, all without pain.

Interesting data has been gathered about this by looking

at people through imaging technology, like MRIs and X-rays. In a systematic review of the literature, researchers looked at 3,110 people who did not have symptoms. Imaging of these people's spines showed that for those under the age of 40, more than 50% had disc degeneration or bulging.[10] Remember, no symptoms for these folks, despite having a change to their tissues that is often considered to be a problematic tissue issue.

In a study on knees of asymptomatic people, 44 people who had no history of knee pain, injury, or bone or joint disease were recruited and their knees were imaged. 43 of the 44 had at least one abnormality in the meniscus tissue. Also of note from that study was that of the 44 studied, 27 had abnormalities in *at least* three of the four regions of the knee. Here again, no symptoms in these folks, despite alterations in their tissues that often get called problematic tissue issues that need attention of some kind.[11]

There are more studies just like these that show the prevalence of abnormalities, tears, and degeneration in tissues, all without pain being present, but the last study I want to share has an interesting spin on it. In this particular study, the researchers gathered a group of elite overhead athletes (over-

10   Brinkjiki et al. (2014) Systematic literature review of imaging features of spinal degeneration in asymptomatic populations *AJNR. American journal of neuroradiology,* 36(4), 811-816. https://doi.org/10.3174/ajnr.A4173

11   Beattie, et al. (2005). Abnormalities identified in the knees of asymptomatic volunteers using peripheral magnetic resonance imaging. *Osteoarthritis and cartilage,* 13(3), 181-186. https://doi.org/10.1016/j.joca.2004.11.001

head athletes are people who play baseball, tennis, volley-ball, and similar sports in which the arm has to travel in an arc overhead regularly) who had no symptoms of shoulder pain, injury, or disease in their dominant arm.

They imaged both the dominant and non-dominant arms of these athletes and found 40% had findings in their dominant shoulder consistent with partial- or full-thickness tears of the rotator cuff. Again, no symptoms. But it gets better. They followed up with these folks five years later to see if shoulder-related symptoms had developed. A grand total of 0% had developed symptoms or problems with their shoulders.[12]

So let's restate this once more: the sensation of pain can emerge due to many factors, some of which are related to the physical status of your tissues, many of which are not related to the physical status of your tissues. Your brain is forming an opinion about a situation and the information it is receiving, and that opinion may or may not correlate a tissue issue with the sensation of pain or vice versa.

Let's look at this through a simple analogy that is used often to explain how a variety of factors can influence if and when you experience pain. Now, bear in mind that nothing in the body is 'just like' something that isn't the body, so analogies are not to be taken literally but rather used as a

---

12   Connor et al. (2003). Magnetic resonance imagine of the asymptomatic shoulder of overhead athletes: a 5 year follow up study. *The American journal of sports medicine*, 31(5), 724-727. https://doi.org/10.1177/03635465030310051501

mental model of what we're talking about with the body.

So: imagine a cup that is filled with each thing you have to deal with each day — maybe for you it's job stress, repetitive movements, worries you have about your back 'going out' on you, a lack of meaningful connection with family or friends, or a lack of physical activity and exercise.

It all gets poured into the one cup, and if the cup overflows, you experience pain. If the decision by your brain to create a painful sensation is a sign that the cup is overflowing, then all the things you're dealing with each day, both in your conscious and subconscious, and the size of your cup, are going to influence if and when that cup overflows. What you can do to avoid spilling the contents of the cup is to either take some things out of the cup, or get a bigger cup to hold it all.

The cup analogy is a simple way to grasp that there are many additional factors beyond an injured tissue that will influence if and when that cup overflows.

Now, let's take it a step further because while a cup is easy to picture in your mind, it also implies more of a linear trajectory of things, whereas your body ecosystem is just that, an ecosystem, and thus, things are constantly in flux and there are multiple signals being responded to at any given time.

CHAPTER 11:

Useful (& Fun) Things You Can Do To Tend To Pain

Several months into healing from my ACL injury, I noticed pain re-emerge in my knee. I hadn't had any pain in two months. None, zero, nada. Then all of a sudden, there was pain. First, I acknowledged that I was experiencing a painful sensation — no hiding from it, no ignoring it and pushing through as if it weren't there.

Acknowledging the current status of things serves you in a few ways. First, if you'll recall, the first step to exploring is to identify your surroundings in the ecosystem in which you find yourself. Second, by acknowledging what you're feeling in your body, you can also clarify to yourself that this is an experience you are having, not something that you are.

Dr. Seth Oberst says, "You are not the pain you feel." This is important because when you begin to identify with something, you tend to make it more ingrained into who you are as a person. And even though pains and injuries can feel dominant at times, they are not an immutable trait of who you are.

In continuing my exploration of the situation, I thought back on my recent days and knew that I hadn't overdone it with workouts, walking, or any other sort of physical activity. And I knew I hadn't had an acute incident that set off a re-injury or anything of that sort. So what was going on here? The context for this piece of painful data in my knee showed up when I thought about the internal signals that could be influencing this. What I *had* experienced in the days leading up to the re-emergence of a painful sensation in my knee was an incredibly stress-inducing situation, and more importantly, my ability to deal with that stressful situation felt similar to drowning in the ocean. That is, I didn't handle it well. I didn't have enough 'room in my cup' and my system seemed to respond by creating a painful sensation in my knee.

I know it can seem a little mind-bending to consider the possibility that while the pain you are experiencing is very real, the cause of it isn't exactly tangible or definitive in the way other things about your existence seem to be. But in opening to the notion that pain can be the response to multiple signals, and that response in and of itself is more of an opinion of your brain, rather than a cold, hard, fact about a situation, you end up creating a lot more opportunities for yourself with regard to how to tend to it.

Remember the Three What's & A Who questioning framework that is part of the Explorer's Mindset: what internal signals and external signals might be contributing to this, what is the opportunity, and who can help?

With my answers to those questions, I was able to select an experiment that I hypothesized would help me both build a bigger cup and assist me in reducing the daily stressors that were going into my cup.

Stop, In The Name Of Pain... (But Not For Good)

We'll get to the experiments I did to resolve my out-of-the-blue knee pain, but first we need to discuss movement as it relates to pain. There's the old eye-rolling joke about a man who goes to the doctor saying he's got a pain in his arm. The doctor asks him what causes the pain and the man replies, "When I do this" and demonstrates the movement that evokes the pain. The doctor replies, "Then stop doing that." In addition to being a real groan of a joke, it's a poor illustration of how to handle moving your body when you're experiencing pain.

When it comes to doing movement that hurts, should you never do it? Do it sometimes? Or should you do it all the time? The fact is that with movement and pain, it is not a simple 'if this = do that' or 'if this = don't do that', but there are some helpful things to know about how movement and pain affect each other that will help you make the right call for you as caretaker of your Unbreakable body.

First, continuing to do movements that are painful may make your brain more likely to create painful sensations. You know how if you practice something enough you'll improve your proficiency at it? Your nervous system follows that practice-improvement curve with everything it does — including becoming more proficient at the process of creating a painful sensation when information is presented in a way that makes your brain associate movement and pain.

Called long-term potentiation, this happens when an existing pathway between two brain cells gets used frequently enough that it becomes 'strengthened', or easier to fire those two brain cells together again. It's what happens when you repeat something enough times that you become more proficient at it — awesome if you're learning how to crawl as a baby, for performing the techniques used in the sport you want to excel at, and for learning another language... less awesome if you're experiencing pain.

When your brain learns to associate a certain movement or movements and pain, you might sense pain even though the injury is long since past. Long-term potentiation is one of numerous factors that appears to be relevant when looking at chronic pain.[13] Not only can the neurons in your brain strengthen to create painful sensations more easily, your tissues and nerves can also become more sensitive to threats and thereby make it easier for them to kick off the process of creating pain.

You've got certain nerve endings that pick up signals from the tissues, called noxious stimuli, that indicate there may be tissue damage and they send that information to your brain for processing and responding to. Those nerve endings can become more sensitive, which you've experienced if you sprained your ankle yesterday and today it's painful just to sit with a pillow pushing into it at the wrong angle. And that's helpful when you're in the middle of an injury, as it acts as a perpetual reminder to you not to move in a particular way when the tissue isn't at full capacity.

But when that increased sensitization becomes prolonged, it can contribute to an acute pain becoming a chronic pain. Given that your brain can learn to associate movement with pain, the notion of pushing through the pain is really a poor suggestion (unless you're being paid to suffer or you're trying out for a high-level military position where the whole point is to outlast someone else's tolerance to suffering). Thankfully, anything your brain can learn and become better at, it

---

13 Bree, Dara. (2019 September 13) *A Causal Role for Long-Term Potentiation in Chronic Pain*. Retrieved from https://www.painresearchforum.org/news/124316-causal-role-long-term-potentiation-chronic-pain

can also un-learn and become less-better at, or rather, it can learn something new and become better at something else that changes the pain-movement association it previously learned. This brings us to the second thing you'll want to know about pain and movement.

Doing movements that are pain-free may help you become able to do more movements that are pain-free. One of the most common things a person does when experiencing a painful sensation is to move less *overall*, and what movements they still do tend to be more cautious and smaller in scope.

This has several impacts, starting first with the impact to quality of life. If you are moving less, you're likely doing fewer of the things you enjoy. This alone can alter your emotional and mental state, and then you add in the fact that you feel stiff, pained, and uncomfortable in your body, it understandably alters your emotional and mental state even more.

Another impact of moving less is that motion assists your body in a wide array of cellular activities, from moving blood and lymph through your body so that nutrients are brought in and waste materials are removed, to building and maintaining the strength and health of soft tissues like muscles and ligaments and hard tissues like bones. And so by removing movement, you're removing a signal to your body that influences a multitude of responses that are relevant for your health and physical fitness.

A simple phrase attributed to physiotherapist, Greg Lehman, regarding the process of healing, takes a complex situation and streamlines it nicely. "Calm stuff down, build stuff up." The phrase is simple but carries a lot of action in it. Whether you're calming tissues down or building them up, what you're actually doing is managing a lot of biochemical and nervous system activity by way of sending particular signals to your body.

The point of calming things down is, in part, to clear noxious stimuli in the area, allow inflammation to do its thing, and to down-regulate the afferent nerve fibers that have sent info to the brain that has influenced the creation of the painful sensation. The point of building things up is to make the tissues that are currently dealing with the issue and the tissues that are related to this issue become stronger and more tolerant to the type of loading you want to put on them through whatever activity you want to do.

And so, when you're experiencing a painful sensation, there are likely a few (or many) movements that feel painful, but there are also likely many that don't feel painful. For example, if your shoulder is bothering you, chances are it hurts in particular motions or positions, but what about all the other motions and positions a shoulder can do? By using your Explorer's Mindset to explore, experiment, and curate, you're able to find the ones that don't hurt and you can then include them in your healing strategy.

By finding movements you can do without pain, you're more likely to resume movements and activities you enjoyed, which can contribute positively to your emotional and mental wellbeing. Finally, by finding movements that don't hurt (including perhaps taking the movement that hurts and finding another way of doing it that doesn't hurt), you're introducing new and different information to your nervous system.

Your brain likes novelty, and something new and different will fire neurons together in a new way, which may lead you to experience your body and the painful sensation in a new way. A fun example of this is something I learned from a physical therapist years ago that he used to help his patients see that pain, or rather, your experience of it, can be influenced simply by doing something different.

If a patient felt pain when turning their neck to look left or right, sometimes he would have them sit on a swivel chair and turn their neck to the side that hurt. Then he'd have them hold their head straight forward and keep their eyes looking forward for as long as they could while they turned the swivel chair — their body turned away while their eyes stayed looking forward. They'd do so without pain, despite the motion being exactly the same as when they'd just turned their head. The only difference was that their body turned first, not their eyes and head. Same, but different. Novelty doesn't have to be radically different for it to be impactful for your brain.

The third thing I want to share with you about movement and pain is that one of the ways your nervous system helps you avoid experiencing pain in the first place is by reducing your range of motion and your ability to move freely with your body. Recall how the two branches of your autonomic nervous system, the 'fight or flight' and 'rest and digest' systems, are perpetually ramping up or down based on the conditions at hand. If your nervous system has become ramped up into that 'fight or flight' sympathetic nervous system response, it's only logical that it would make your body more ready to face whatever stressful thing you're clearly facing.

From Dr. Seth Oberst: "When stressed and rigid, we lose the ability to rotate our joints because they are no longer centered in the socket as our brains tighten the joints to protect from injury during a threatening experience."

In addition to that, your brain will increase muscle tone throughout your body and unfortunately, this is not the kind of 'muscle tone' that comes to mind when you think of having toned biceps and thighs. This type of muscle tone is about resting tension, or stiffness, of the muscles, and when you've got increased muscle tone it makes you more ready to fight or flee, but it can also make you feel more stiff, rigid, tense, and uncomfortable. So it's possible that the aches and pains you feel in your body may very well have been born out of your nervous system just trying to protect you from a perceived threat.

But you don't have to wait until you're living that no-stress life to begin feeling and moving better. You can use your Explorer's Mindset to explore the current environment of your body ecosystem, collect data that informs you about what your body ecosystem is currently dealing with, select an experiment that is a good match for the environment in which you are experimenting, and over time, curate various signals that work best for the different environments your body ecosystem will shift through as you go through life.

Here's an example to illustrate this: exercise (or any signal you want to send to your body, for that matter) is not a one-dimensional static thing that can only be applied in one exact way. For instance, exercise can be done at a low intensity, a high intensity, or at any of the intensities between 'low' and 'high'. It can also be done at various frequencies and for various durations. It can include more or fewer rest breaks. It can be done in all sorts of styles and sequences. And whether or not it makes you feel better and stronger in your body, or worse and more stiff has to do, in part, with whether the way you're doing it aligns with what your body ecosystem is able to currently handle.

If the realities of life right now mean that your body ecosystem is starting from a place of stress, tension, and stiffness, then you're not likely to have the same capacity, readiness, and recovery ability as someone who is not starting from that place. By exploring and collecting data about your current environment, you're able to take the signal of 'exercise' and tailor it to suit the environment you're currently in. And even if you decide not to tailor the exercise signal to match your current environment, but rather go hard with exercise because that's how the workout program was written, even if your body feels like it's breaking down in the process, that too is a useful experiment.

Over time, you'll do enough experiments to find the limits of what your body ecosystem can tolerate and respond to favorably when it is in various states of stress. By curating the responses to these experiments, you'll become the foremost expert in knowing how to adapt any exercise program you decide to partake in so that it perfectly fits what your body ecosystem will respond most favorably to right now.

Let's go back now to that knee pain that re-emerged after I'd been pain-free for months, because this is likely to happen to you as well at some point. You'll be going along, doing great at tending to your body so it feels good, strong, and pain-free, and then — boom — seemingly out of nowhere an ache, a pain, or some kind of irritating issue will emerge. It doesn't mean that you've finally hit that point where it's 'too late', it simply means that your body is letting you know that something about the signals you're sending may be not working as you'd prefer and some new or varied signals may be in order.

As I went through the Three What's & A Who questioning framework, I quickly zeroed in on that stressful event and how I responded to it. Having been on my journey of becoming Unbreakable for so long by this point, I had developed enough wisdom to know that it wasn't likely to be movement, sleep, or food that was contributing to the response of knee pain, but rather, that it was most likely this particularly stressful situation that was doing it.

Of course, as an Unbreakable human you're always willing to revisit other signals if experiments with the ones you chose to focus on don't give you the outcomes you were hoping for. With the stressful event and my stress response in my sights, I selected two experiments, the first being to resume a mindfulness practice called "Open Focus"[14] that I'd let slide over the last year. It wasn't that I thought I might zen my way to being pain-free, but rather, this type of mindfulness practice can alter the way you focus, which can alter your brainwaves so that you can relate to pain in a new way.

And the second experiment was to incorporate at least ten minutes of play into every day. Yes, play, the thing you did when you were a kid. Like the mindfulness practice, there's neat science in there[15] that can positively impact how you experience and relate to pain. Let's look into both of these more closely…

Brainwaves, Play, & Pain

As your brain processes and synthesizes information, masses of neurons are firing together in your brain, which produces synchronized electrical pulses known as brainwaves. You have several types of brainwaves and they influence many

---

14   Fehmi and Shor (2018 July19) *Open Focus*. Retrieved from https://openfocus.com/

15   He et al., (2015). Therapeutic play intervention on children's perioperative anxiety, negative emotional manifestation and postoperative pain: a randomized controlled trial. *Journal of advanced nursing*, 71(5), 1032-1043. https://doi.org/10.1111/jan.12608

things, including your ability to learn something new and how you experience pain.

In the 1960's, Dr. Les Fehmi, who is a world-renowned leader in the field of neurofeedback, was trying hard to train his brain to produce more alpha brain waves. Brainwaves are broken down into five main frequencies: alpha, beta, delta, gamma, and theta. Each frequency correlates with different behaviors in your brain. For instance, delta waves occur during sleep while beta waves occur when you are awake, alert, and doing most of your tasks during your day. Your brain shifts to alpha waves, the kind Fehmi was trying to produce, when you are relaxed and calm yet still alert — a bit like how you might feel during meditation or when in a 'flow state' while doing something. Fehmi was in the lab with an EEG machine hooked up to his scalp to read his brain's waves, trying to get his brain to make more alpha waves. He tried and tried to induce that relaxed sort of state… but he kept failing miserably.

As he says in his book, *Dissolving Pain,* he just couldn't do it and gave up.[16] To his surprise, as soon he gave up, his alpha waves increased. As he put it, "It was the letting go of effort" that finally produced the alpha waves. He couldn't get to the relaxed alpha brain wave state by trying harder and focusing more intently, and in fact, the way he was using

16   Fehmi and Robbins (2010) *Dissolving Pain: Simple Brain-Training Exercises for Overcoming Chronic Pain.* Boulder, Colorado, USA: Trumpeter Books

his attention was hindering his ability to accomplish it.

So Fehmi was in his lab and he'd achieved a state of relaxation by stopping his try-hard efforts — who cares? Well, over the next few days he reported a number of positive changes, including that the tone of his muscles had softened, that he felt less irritable and anxious, and that the tension and pain he'd been experiencing had melted away. As it turned out, if your intention is to get rid of pain and/or learn something new, the state of your brainwaves will have an impact on how successful you are.

Dr. Fehmi has spent more than forty years studying how a person's directed attention — their focus, influences their experience of pain. And what he found was that there are several types of focus, some of which make it more difficult to experience a lessening or a resolving of pain and others which make it easier to do so. In addition, Fehmi found that being able to switch between different types of focus (what he called 'flexible attention') was also an important factor in how a brain manages painful sensations.

When you hear the words 'focus' or 'attention', you might think of studying for an exam or driving on an icy highway at night. These are indeed experiences that require a certain type of attention, namely a narrow-objective focus, but there are also several other ways of focusing on things according to how Fehmi categorizes things.

The styles of attention or focus are: narrow attention, which creates a hyper-focus on one thing at the exclusion of everything else in the environment, objective attention, which creates separation between the observer and the thing being observed, immersed attention, which as the name suggests occurs when you're completely 'in the zone' and operating effortlessly, and diffuse attention, which creates a softer sense of focus that takes in everything without focusing intently on any one thing.

Most of your daily life is likely spent using narrow-objective focus — not just with sight but with all the senses — and it's understandable. The beta brainwaves you use in narrow-objective focus allow you to process things quickly, they enhance your sense of alertness, and they improve your reasoning and critical thinking. However, this type of focus also comes at a cost. It keeps you shifted more into your sympathetic 'fight or flight' nervous system. You already know that being perpetually stuck in either branch of the autonomic nervous system can become an issue, and being more ramped up into the sympathetic response means you're less likely to be in a state of calm ease, which can make it more difficult to resolve pain. It can also make it more difficult to fully sense your surroundings, take a full breath, or alter the tonicity of your muscles since they will have greater tonicity, or tension, when you are in your fight or flight response.

Not to mention the widespread health impacts of being in a chronically stressed state, such as an increased risk of coronary heart disease, diabetes, hypertension, high cholesterol, sleep issues, depression and anxiety issues, to name just a few.

On top of narrow-objective attention keeping you stuck in the sympathetic nervous system, Fehmi found that using narrow-objective focus with an existing painful sensation can also make that painful sensation feel worse and last longer. Examples of this include focusing intently on the area that is hurting, thinking about how it doesn't feel good, worrying that something serious might be wrong, and focusing intensely on getting rid of the sensation.

And if you read that and thought, "Oh, you mean like how I fixate on pain when I'm in it?" Yes, exactly. In doing so, you end up in a roundabout situation. You focus intently on the pain, that narrow focus increases your muscle tension, ramps up your sympathetic nervous system, and makes your brain less effective at processing pain signals, making it more reactive and hypersensitive, so you become more sensitive to pain, more aware of it, more rigid about it, more stressed about it, more stuck in it, and on round you go.

You'd think that if that's the case with narrow-objective focus, then perhaps doing the opposite would be better: completely ignoring the pain, learning to distract and distance yourself from it. But it turns out, that's not the ticket either, as this too is a form of narrow-objective focus. Here, rather than narrowing your focus on the painful sensation, you're narrowing your focus on something else, which Fehmi says teaches your system to repress pain.

Instead, he found that learning to broaden and soften your focus is more conducive to experiencing a lessening or resolving of the painful sensation. When you broaden your focus to be more diffuse and immersive, which Fehmi calls "open focus", the painful sensation becomes just one thing in a whole landscape of things, thereby taking it from being the only thing you can think about to being one thing amongst a lot of other things.

Or put another way, instead of the painful sensation being one hundred percent of what you're aware of, it becomes ten per cent or some similar small percentage, which means the majority of your awareness is not consumed by the painful sensation. Along with the focus shift, your nervous system, and thus your whole body, gets the chance to move out of the ramped-up state and into a state where more learning and healing can occur.

It's also worth mentioning here that how you focus your attention on your body is not limited to when you experience pain or injury. If you have disliked parts of your body at any point in your life, or been told parts of you were not attractive or good enough, you may start to hyper-focus on them: you always want to change them or are disappointed that they are not what you want them to be, or you may shut them out entirely, as they are a source of discomfort for you.

If you have beliefs that your shoulder is 'always an issue' or that your left side is 'always your bad side', these thoughts may make you see yourself in an adversarial relationship with your body, or with parts of your body on the opposing team to yourself. You might even see yourself as a collection of parts, rather than as a whole person. And if you've ever been so motivated to accomplish something that you do it despite your body clearly telling you that it's not holding up, you may realize that when you really look at how you're using your attention, you only have one way to use it at this point in time. Even if you have not experienced one of these examples of focusing on your body, living in the modern world tends to shift you into narrow-objective focus with minimal opportunity to shift out of it unless you are proactive about doing so.

Dr. Fehmi has many great experiments in his books that you can do to shift into an alpha brainwave state but for now, here's a simple example of his most basic Open Focus meditation: pause and allow your awareness to expand from the words on this page or screen to include both the words you're looking at and the spaces between the words.

Can you let the spaces between the words have as much of your attention as the words themselves?

Can you then let your gaze expand to include the words on the page, the spaces between the words, and whatever is on the left and right sides of the page or screen?

Softening your eyes so you're gazing rather than staring can help you start to get this. Give yourself a few moments to experience this and see how you do with it.

Initially, it may feel impossible to continue registering what is on the page while expanding your awareness so that your focus includes what you're reading and other things in your field of vision. But eventually you'll get the hang of it and you might notice that almost as soon as you shift your focus, you might take a deeper breath, which causes you to realize you weren't taking deep and full breaths before.

Consider that if you didn't notice that you weren't taking full breaths, there might be others things missing from your noticing. The old saying goes "You don't know what you don't know" and I'd add to it, "You don't notice what you don't notice."

Being able to shift your brainwave state when you're experiencing a painful sensation is not just valuable for changing your experience of the pain, although that's powerful in and of itself. You also begin to cultivate an enhanced form of exploring, going from noticing only the most obvious aspects of your inner and outer environment to being able to notice the more subtle aspects that had previously slipped by your radar.

The first time I learned to shift into more of an alpha state with my brainwaves, I almost didn't believe what I was experiencing. The pain I felt got quiet, as if it wasn't taking up so much space within me. It got smaller and felt less tense, and I felt aware of much more of myself and my surroundings now, and in turn, the painful sensation felt like just a tiny piece of it all.

That dovetailed nicely with the second experiment I ran concurrently with the mindfulness experiment, to incorporate ten minutes of play into my day. Play shouldn't need an explanation since it's literally just free play like you did as a kid, but adults often struggle to conceptualize what free play looks like at this stage of life.

You're no longer a child who goes out to play on the swingset, or who rounds up the neighborhood kids for a game. My childhood friends and I loved to play a game called "throw the ball over the telephone pole wire and whoever catches it gets to go next." Simpler times, to be sure. Whatever you played as a kid, it was likely woven with a sense of mindless immersiveness that both kept your attention easily and made you forget about everything else, like getting home in time for dinner.

Unfortunately, as you get older, any sort of movement you do is for a particular end goal with particular parameters around it, like exercising for thirty minutes three times a week and doing movements A, B, C, and D, each with their own particular technique for ten reps each. There's nothing wrong with that kind of movement, in fact, it's a part of the bedrock of building muscles, bones, and fitness in your body. But it's different from play, and whether healing aches or pains or not, adults would likely do well to have more play in their life.

The structure of free play is that there is no structure, and while it could look like going outside to play some imagination-based game or hopping on the swingset at the park, it can also be a lot simpler than that. Imagine sitting on the couch or on the floor, or even laying in a bed if you prefer to start there, and for the next ten minutes you're going to just move your limbs in whatever random way you think of.

- How many different ways can you sit up from a laying down position?
- How many different ways can you move your spine?
- How many different movements of your limbs and joints can you string together so you flow from one thing to the next?
- If using a prop makes you feel more at ease, grab a throw pillow and start tossing it up and down seeing if you can catch it in different ways... with two hands, with one, higher toss, twisting toss, and so on. How many ways can you find to interact with the pillow?

These are just a few simple examples and questions you can use to start exploring free play in its most simple form — exploration without any expectation. Allow yourself to be immersed in exploring the movements and your body as you move it. By doing so, you increase the potential of tapping into a state of flow.

"A flow state is defined as the mental state in which a person performing some activity is fully immersed in a feeling of energized focus, full involvement, and enjoyment in the process of the activity."[17] It is characterized by a shift into a

17 Csikszentmihalyi, M. (2004, February). *Flow, the secret to happiness.* [Video]. TED Conferences. https://www.ted.com/talks/mihaly_csikszentmihalyi_flow_the_secret_to_happiness

brainwave state that borders between alpha and theta, and it's not just for elite athletes or people at the peak of their expertise in their profession.

Flow state is for everyone, and by remembering how to play you're tapping into one of the many ways there is to achieve a flow state. It might feel strange at first, to have no rules, but try to remember that ten-year old You would have given anything to have no rules.

Over the course of the next week or so, I kept up my commitment to do the experiments each day, and my knee pain subsided and disappeared. I ended up keeping up the mindfulness and play for quite some time simply because I enjoyed how it made me feel, and have since saved those two actions in my Unbreakable Field Journal as good options to revisit should I find myself in a similar situation in the future.

But how did I know that it was those things that made my knee feel better? What if it was just random chance? Well, it could have been living life waiting for random chance to happen is not a strategy that aligns with my personal vision for becoming Unbreakable. You'll have to decide for yourself if it aligns with your vision, but whether it does or not, you'll always learn more when you participate in the process than if you sit on the sidelines. Besides, this is one of the beautiful aspects of choosing to use an Explorer's Mindset to take care of your Unbreakable body — the exploring, experimenting, and curating never ends.

Thus, if I have the knee pain sensation again in the future

and I try the same two experiments again, but this time they don't seem to impact the pain in my knee the same way, I've learned something new and gained more perspective on me, my knee, and the inner and outer environments of my body ecosystem. When you don't get the outcome you expected based on previous outcomes, you get the opportunity to see the situation from another perspective and to ask more and better questions.

What If You Still Have Pain?

If you're experiencing something painful, unpleasant, or disruptive — and let's be real here, it's usually all three at once — all you want is for it to go away. This painful disruption is hampering your life, it's keeping you from doing the things you want to do, it's exhausting you, and it's probably costing you on all fronts. You aren't physically capable of doing the things you most enjoy and the gap between where you are and where you want to be feels large. It's only natural that you might begin to ruminate on thoughts like 'what if this never goes away?' So let's face the big, hairy, 'what if' worry head on.

When I was healing that ACL injury, I couldn't do any of the activities I loved for months. I had days where I felt confident and optimistic about my future. Those tended to also be the days when I noticed progress in my rehabilitation drills or in my pain level. I also had days when I cried over an imagined future where my ability to access the outdoors

— something that is vital to my wellbeing and my notion of who I am as a person — felt like it was going to be permanently altered.

On those tough days, I worried that I wouldn't be able to hike off deep into the mountains, which led to worrying that I'd never get to interact with nature in the ways I relished, which led to worrying that I'd lose a major part of who I feel myself to be at my core. When I really looked closely at my 'what if' worries, I realized I wasn't worried about 'what if' regarding activities, I was asking, "What if I can't be *me* anymore because of this injury?"

As soon as I realized that, I felt a deeper sense of understanding myself, and was able to take on the role of comforting myself and helping myself to rationally navigate through that deeper worry. To find out if there's something deeper (and there's almost *always* something deeper) in your 'what if' worries, use your Explorer's Mindset on those worries, with a focus particularly on using curious compassion to explore into it.

Remember that when you collect data you're also going to end up collecting stories that are tethered to that data, and emotions about the stories and the data? Pick up that 'what if' worry and see what stories you have that are linked to the 'what if'. Explore under the emotion of worry to see what other emotions are there as well. Chances are, all those stories and emotions are there for a reason; remember that your body is always responding to something. Use experiments to take these charged stories and emotions and see if you can rework them in such a way as to make them more helpful while reducing the grip they have on you.

But what if your 'what if' worry becomes reality and the pain never leaves? That will be true for some people. Life-altering situations happen, issues that were disruptive can become debilitating, and sometimes those problems that you reframed as areas of opportunity stick around long enough that you seriously wonder if you've exhausted all opportunities and this has become a permanent part of your existence. And if that is where you find yourself, let's just call it out right now: that sucks.

You're going to have to find your path forward as an Unbreakable human, just as you have been up to this point. Consider allowing yourself to mourn, to feel angry, and to feel the full range of whatever you're feeling. Know that you are not alone and it might be helpful to talk to someone. Start the process of envisioning what your future will look like, but don't feel like you have to have it all figured out right now. Keep on being an excellent caretaker of your Unbreakable body in whatever way you can.

Now that you know that pain can emerge due to a multitude of factors, and that pain can be present without tissue damage, and tissue damage can be present without pain, we can move into talking about building your body's tissues so that you feel how you want to feel and can move how you want to move.

CHAPTER 12:

How Do Tissues Change?

Tissues in your body — whether muscle tissue, connective tissue, bone tissue, joint capsule tissue, or any other tissue in your body — tend to feel how you want them to feel, and make you capable of doing all you want to do, when they are well-constructed and well-functioning. And tissues become well-constructed and well-functioning when they are signaled to regularly about what they should respond to. And the conversation your tissues respond most favorably to is that of forces.

Forces range from gravity pressing down on you at all

times, to movements you do, positions you assume, cardio-vascular activity, and even the type of shoes and clothing you wear are forces on your body. Whether it's through a workout or your daily life, force is a constant signal your body is responding to.

Your body's tissues will respond to the signal of 'force' by improving their function and capacity to handle those forces better in the future. The opposite of this is true as well. When your tissues do not experience forces, the tissue's function becomes less efficient and its capacity decreases.

Our understanding of forces, in this context, began in the nineteenth century, with a man named Julius Wolff. He was a surgeon and anatomist, and he postulated a law (which became known as Wolff's Law) that states that "the bone in a healthy person or animal will adapt to the loads under which it is placed." [18] He found that if loading on a particular bone increases, the bone will remodel itself over time to become stronger to resist that sort of loading. The inverse of this is true as well. If loading on a bone decreases, the bone will become weaker and less dense.

You've seen this when a person develops osteoporosis. You naturally lose bone density as you age, in part because the cellular processes by which new bone is made slow down. But in addition to that, the likelihood increases that you'll do less weight-bearing activity as you get older. And less weight-

---

18   Wolff J. (1986). *The law of bone Remodelling.* Berlin, Germany: Springer-Verlag

bearing activity (signal!) means less forces for bones to respond to, which means less dense bones. It's the inverse of Wolff's Law in action. This is one reason why older adults (or any person who wants denser bones) are strongly encouraged to do weight training and weight-bearing activities. Bone remodeling may slow down over time, but you can exert your conscious influence on that process by intentionally sending signals that cause your bones to respond by becoming denser and thereby offset the natural process of aging bones.

What Wolff figured out was that loading on the bone is a form of communication to the cells and non-cellular tissue that makes up the bone. The communication from the forces on the bones tells the cells of the bone what should happen to make the bone more tolerant of that kind of loading. When you send a signal by way of a force placed on the bone, the bone responds by increasing its tolerance to that force, thereby increasing its capacity.

Another man, an orthopedic surgeon named Henry Gassett Davis, developed another law that follows on from Wolff's, called Davis's Law. This law is used to describe how soft tissue models itself in response to imposed demands and follows the same concept of communication that bone cells respond to.

Specifically, Davis's Law states that soft tissue heals according to the manner in which it is mechanically stressed. Mechanical stressors are forces that are being placed on the tissues through pressure and motion. As with a bone, when you send a signal by way of a force placed on the soft tissue, such as by way of a movement or muscle contraction, the soft tissue responds by increasing its tolerance to that force, thereby increasing its capacity. So if you want stronger, better tissues, you'll need to signal to your tissues via forces, of which movement is a big one, so that the tissues can respond by becoming more tolerant, and thus, stronger and better.

The way the tissues become more tolerant of forces it experiences is by organizing the microscopic cellular components of the tissue in such a way that those cellular components actually reorganize and realign themselves in the same direction as the directional force that was placed on the tissue. Think of it like this, if you are in charge of a group of people and your group needs to accomplish a task, the first thing you'd want to do is organize everybody so that they know your plan for how the group will work together to accomplish the task. What you wouldn't want is five people doing one thing, a few others twiddling their thumbs over in the corner, and the rest all doing random things. On a microscopic level, your body is doing a similar "let's all get organized so we can accomplish the task" sort of thing when it experiences forces on tissues. To demonstrate this, here's an experiment researchers did using liquid and some lab-grown cells. The researchers made note that when they grew cells they were going to use for this test, the stress fibers (which are one of the microscopic cellular components of cells and who play a central role in force transmission, as well as in cell movement, and many other tasks) were oriented randomly with some fibers pointing one way, others pointing another.

The researchers then sent fluid flowing across the top of the cells. The sheer stress of the fluid flowing in one direction was a force on the cells, causing the cells to elongate and orient the fibers within them in the direction of the flow. But this didn't happen if they just sent a droplet or two of water flowing over top of these cells. The ongoing signal of the directional force of the water factored into how those cells and fibers responded.

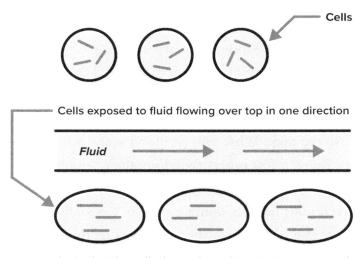

Cells

Cells exposed to fluid flowing over top in one direction

Fluid

(note that the cells themselves elongate to a more oval shape and the fibers all orient the same way)

The directional force of the water flowing made the cells and fibers orient themselves in the same direction, and the forces you exert on your body will cultivate a similar response in your tissues. Yes, the fibers that are in your cells of your tissues will reorganize and align themselves based on the forces they experience similar to how the fibers in the lab experiment did. These fibers within your tissues are important for a variety of things, including sensing forces and for cellular mechanics, and it appears that fibers oriented in a more organized fashion will withstand and transmit forces better in the future, as well as help with long-term tissue remodeling. So more organized and aligned fibers means more, better, tissues that will respond more favorably to forces (ie, movements and positions) in the future.

When those forces on the tissues are consistent, specific, and intentional, you make the tissue stronger so it can tolerate those particular forces better. Here the word 'stronger' doesn't just imply muscular strength either (although consistent, specific, intentional, forces do indeed increase the strength of the muscle). With regard to your tissues, 'stronger' also means that a bone will become denser, skin tissue will become thicker (as with calluses), ligaments and tendons will become thicker and more resilient to forces placed on them, and cartilage will become denser. Forces are at the root of all of the signals you send to build the tissues of your body so they can do the things you want them to do, and so you can build tissues that are as resilient and resistant to aches and pains as you'd like.

Wolff and Davis both pointed out that forces don't just impact one tissue in your body. And thankfully so, because nobody has time to have a one-on-one meeting with every tissue of your body every single week. It turns out that when a force is sent to a particular tissue, the tissues in the surrounding area — and some tissues that are much further away — can also 'hear' and respond to the force.

This happens thanks to something called the extracellular matrix (ECM for short). The ECM is essential in a number of processes — here are just a few: tissue growth, wound healing, the expression of the DNA within a cell, scar formation, and cell organization within the tissue. And the ECM facilitates cell-to-cell communication: cells 'talk' to each other through the ECM within which they live, and one of the ways they do this is by sensing tension changes in the ECM. These tension changes occur when forces are placed on the tissues. For instance, a muscle contraction generates a force for the muscle tissue, but it also generates a force for the tendons that attach the muscle to the bone, for the bone itself, for the joints on either end of the bone, and for other tissues in the area of where the force was applied.

An example is your biceps muscle in your arm. Find an object with some weight to it, like a cooking pan, and hold it in your hand with your elbow bent. The biceps muscle is contracting and generating enough force for you to be able to hold the cooking pan up. That force from the muscle contraction is spreading to the biceps tendons that connect the biceps to the lower arm bone and the shoulder. The force of the contraction continues through to your bones where the tendons attach, and thus the tendons and bones get stronger too because of the force you created by contracting your biceps muscle. On top of that, the force generated by your biceps will also spread out to your forearm, hand, and shoulder muscles, too.

This is because when it comes to your body, the different types of tissue do not have a distinct separation from one to another, as if you get to a point along the muscle where there's a sign saying "you are now leaving Muscleville city limits." Instead, the composition of the extracellular matrix of muscle begins to change and at some point in the tissue, it becomes something else.

Muscle becomes tendon, ligament becomes bone, 'this thing' becomes 'that thing'. Connective tissue in one area flows into and becomes the connective tissue in another area, and my favorite quote from Thomas Myers, author of *Anatomy Trains*, sums it up: "We do not have 600 muscles, but instead we have one muscle in 600 pockets."[19] That is to say, all our muscles are connected, and because they are all connected to so many other tissues in our body, forces felt in one area of tissue will be felt in other areas of tissue as well.

Sending signals by placing forces on your tissues will create stronger tissues now and can positively impact how your tissues remodel themselves over the long-term. As cells

19 Myers, T. (2014). *Anatomy Trains: Myofascial Meridians for Manual and Movement Therapists 3rd Edition*. London, England: Churchill Livingstone

turn over, they pass along information about how to operate to the new cells that will replace them. So if the old cells are organized and aligned to tolerate certain forces, they'll pass that information along to the new cells. Isn't it nice to know that you won't have to start from scratch with the upgrade process for each and every new cell that shows up?

Of course, this doesn't mean you only have to work on your tissue once and then never think about it again. I think you probably know that doing something once doesn't create the same results as doing something regularly, and that doing something once a year doesn't create the same results as doing something three times a week. I really wish that practicing Spanish once was enough for me to speak it fluently, but it's not. My brain will absolutely respond to the novel experience if I only practice it once, but if my end goal is to know how to fluently speak the language, I will need to signal that to my brain more regularly through ongoing practice.

The same is true for your body. Your body will respond to novel stimuli, but not in the same way as it will respond to the repeated exposure to specific, intentional, repetitive forces. Most folks hear the phrase 'specific, intentional, repetitive forces' and think 'exercise'. And while exercise is a form of force on your tissues which can be highly beneficial, it is often a very narrow collection of movements compared to all of the movements your body is capable of making, and is also usually a very tiny amount of time in your day compared to the amount of time in your day that is not spent exercising.

Think of exercise or physical training as the conscious, controlled environment where you can practice, be particular, and train specific things, and think of the rest of your life as the unconscious, uncontrolled environment where you need to be ready to respond in a nearly infinite number of ways without a moment's notice.

So while it's valuable to use your conscious, controlled, training time to move your body in a variety of ways, it's still going to only be a drop in the bucket of ways the real world invites you to move. The ways in which you can include movement in your life are only hindered by your imagination. To help your imagination get going, I included a bonus with this book that guides you through a sequence of movements that help you explore how your body is made to move. You'll find that movement sequence at: www.theunbreakablebody.com/book-bonus/

Translate That Please!

You know now that forces are at the root of the Signal/Response Principle, which your body is engaged in every single day. Pause now and take a little mental meander through your day so far, and notice what forces have been a part of your day. Here's mine as an example:

- The position I slept in
- The position I stood in as I made my coffee
- The sitting cross-legged on the floor position I always

assume while enjoying the first half of my cup of coffee
- The five minutes of breath-based activities I did to help my body position itself and find the respiratory mechanics I'd like my body to use all day today
- The positions I moved through as I did my strength workout before work
- The position I'm sitting in at my desk...

Later today, my list of forces will include the walk I take, the shoes I wear, and even the work pants I put on to go work in the yard which are a stiff material that make them great for doing manual labor but not great for trying to squat down the way I normally would — and thus, the sort of modified awkward squat I do in them is also a force on my body.

What about you? What forces have you signaled to your body with so far today?

Now, we'd be here for years if we tried to list every single force that every single human is responding to every single day. What I'm going to give you instead is a guide to the common force types most of us experience and what they communicate to your body. With these, you can make a practically infinite number of selections with forces to communicate with your body about how you want it to respond.

1) **When you communicate a certain amount of force:**

The weight of something — the weight of your child when you pick them up and carry them on your shoulders at the park, the weight of a dumbbell you use in a workout, the shopping you carry in from the car.

What that translates to for your body:

"Manage this force by contracting your muscles and connective tissues, and moving your joints accordingly, to disperse the forces most effectively across your body."

2) **When you communicate a certain amount of force at a certain frequency:**

So you've lifted the weight of your child, a dumbbell, or the shopping, but did you engage with that amount of force once, or was it on regular occasion?

What that translates to for your body:

When the force is done frequently and consistently: "Improve your ability to contract and move so that you can manage this force better in the future."

When the force is done infrequently and inconsistently: "This is novel so do your best here even though you're not trained for this."

3) **When you communicate the direction that a force is coming from or going to:**

This one might be confusing, so here's an example: picture a basketball player who is running up and down the court during their game. They're looking strong and fit, that is, until they roll their ankle as they pivoted around an opponent. Now they're laying on the ground with a sprained ankle. What happened? They looked strong and fit — and they were! — until their ankle tissues experienced the force of their bodyweight moving in a new direction when their ankle rolled to the side. It's a bit simplistic but let's think of the forces going through the ankle as the player ran the court as going up and down, from the ground up into the body and back down into the ground again. When the player's ankle rolled to the side, all of a sudden the direction of force changed as the outer ankle tissues got stretched as the bodyweight was no longer was well-stacked from ground up through the body.

Direction is a part of every force your body is presented with and responds to. And different directions of force are different. In order to make tissues that are resilient and resistant to as many different kinds of forces as possible, it pays to teach them how to do so by exposing your tissues to a multitude of forces that come from a multitude of directions. Injuries often happen when tissues meet forces they weren't prepared for.

What that translates to for your body:

"Organize your joints, muscles, and connective tissues, so that they can flex in a way that manages this particular line of tension better, and get into this position more easily and tolerate it better in the future."

4) **When you communicate a particular force for an extended period of time, either continuously or repeatedly.**

A continuous force for an extended length of time doesn't have to mean forever, and it doesn't even have to mean 'a long time' on a grand scale. If you use one hand to lift a cast iron pan full of steaming hot food, you're not likely to be holding it for very long. Cast iron pans, for most people, are quite heavy and cumbersome to lift — unless you communicate with your body that it should become more capable of managing that particular force.

Holding the pan without dropping it or straining your wrist might mean that fifteen seconds constitutes a 'continuous force'. Going for a long-distance bike ride, carrying a heavy pack on a backpacking trip for eight hours a day, or spending all weekend raking up all the leaves that have fallen in your backyard constitute more of a repetitive force.

What that translates to for your body:
"Build your capacity to contract and move all these parts so that you can manage a greater volume of this force over a longer duration of time."

5) **When you communicate that you are regularly moving your joint through a certain range of motion.**

Range of motion is the measure of how much movement a particular joint has. You have two ranges of motion: passive and active.

What that translates to for your body:

"This particular range of motion is being used consistently, please maintain the components of this area, all the way down to the cellular bits that make up the tissues here, that are moving and flexing when this motion occurs."

Now, these are all particulars about forces that can make your body more capable of handling those forces in the future. And as I mentioned earlier, there's a flip side here where a lack of forces make you *less* capable of withstanding a force in the future. Most folks think of this in relation to muscle strength — say, if you wear a cast for a period of time the immobilized muscles will become weaker, or if you stop exercising the fitness gains you made will eventually dissipate.

And indeed, losing muscle mass and strength are important factors in overall health. Loss of muscle mass and strength as you age is predictive of a shorter lifespan, and worse recovery after injury or surgery. But these are not the only things you can lose if you don't communicate with your body through forces. How your joints feel and how many degrees of motion they have available to them is also impacted by the forces your joints experience.

Joints are where your bones meet each other — an obvious one is your knee joint, where your femur meets your tibia and your patella. Your muscles will cross your joints, and as such, when you contract your muscles those contractions will cause the joint to move. They do this so automatically and effortlessly that you likely rarely think about it... until they start doing it a bit less effortlessly.

You might begin noticing stiffness, pain, grinding or clicking sensations when you move your joint, or your joints simply won't allow you to move as you wish. When you don't communicate to your joints that you are using their full range of motion, the tissues and cellular components that make them up don't get the memo that they should prioritize maintenance of those tissues.

Because your body is constantly prioritizing and de-prioritizing where it should focus its efforts to maintain and build, if you do not indicate that maintaining that range of motion is a priority, the range will eventually shrink. Knowing this, are you starting to wonder if your stiff knees or inflexible hips are really something that's just a part of who you are, or if they became that way because of the lack of signals (and thus, a lack of forces) they received?

Forces are a conversation you're having with your body and its tissues — all the way down to the cells that make up those tissues — every single moment of every single day. Simply by creating more ways in which you move through your day, you create more communication for your tissues to respond to. Exercise is one valuable process for communicating to your body's tissues through forces, but remember that your daily life is also chock-full of ways to signal to your body through forces:

- Stand instead of sit
- Sit on the floor instead of in a chair
- Sit differently in your chair if you can't sit on the floor yet
- Carry your bag on the other shoulder
- Carry it in your hand instead of on your shoulder
- Walk more
- Swing your arms more when you walk
- Take a short break to move your body after periods of sitting
- If you pick your foot up and put it on a higher surface to tie your shoes, see if you can squat down and tie your shoes while your foot's on the floor
- If you catch yourself holding a lot of tension in your shoulders, arms, and jaw, as you're sitting working on your computer, pause and take a deep breath and let that tension go for a bit

Start making those forces of everyday life work even more in your favor. As the caretaker of your body ecosystem, you can cultivate opportunities to communicate with your body through forces all throughout your day. You can notice the responses your body is making currently, collect some data about what you're noticing, perhaps learn something about the particular data you've collected, then try an experiment where you alter the forces your body is receiving, and note the outcomes that occur. If you like the response you're getting, you can keep going. If you don't, you can use that information to inform how you might adjust the conversation you're having with your body and try again.

This doesn't mean you have to turn your entire life into an experiment like some biohacker, but your entire life is an opportunity for experiment. If you're motivated to make your body feel and move better, and you would like to maintain or even improve that as time goes on, if your vision of being Unbreakable includes doing fun things with your body till your last day on this Earth, if you desire to feel vibrant and youthful (even after age 40, or 60, or 80), then you need to become an active participant in the conversation of forces that you're having with your body.

Truly, one of the biggest 'bang for your buck' actions you can take is to start communicating with your body through the intentional forces you place on your body. When you encourage your cells to organize along the line of stress being imparted from specific directional forces, you make the cells, and thus the tissues, stronger and more effective in their ability to manage that particular force or stress in the future. And when you build better tissues, you make it more likely that you'll feel great in your body as well.

This is true even with tissues that have had no consistent directional force up to this point. If you've never known that managing the forces you place on your body can impact how your body feels, now you do. That is to say, it's never too late to start. Sending these specific directional forces is like a tissue 'upgrade', and of all the things you can upgrade in this world — seats on the plane, your cable TV package, the streaming service that offers the 'no ads' premium level — one of the most impactful things you can upgrade is your tissue.

Now, I have mentioned a few times that forces influence how you feel, how you heal, how you move, and what you can do. It's common to think that the forces used for *feeling* and *healing* are different from the forces used for *moving* and *doing*. In reality, they are two sides of the same coin, as you'll see in the next chapter. You're going to learn how to build your body to be strong and capable by looking at what happens when you sustain an injury.

CHAPTER 13:

How Do Injuries Happen?

We've just looked at how forces on your body's tissues communicate to your body about how to make tissues that feel and function better for you. Now that you know that, we can look at what happens when tissues aren't as strong as we'd like them to be and an injury occurs. Understanding both how tissues are formed and how tissues break down in an injury will help you put the whole tissue-building equation together.

A quick note before we dive in: remember that we learned a few chapters back that there are many aspects which can contribute to whether or not you feel pain, *and* that it's possible to feel pain without having any tissue damage and tissue damage without pain. What we're going to focus on now is what is happening when you sustain some level of tissue damage, because understanding that will help you make yourself more resistant to that sort of thing in the future.

How Much Can Your Body Tolerate Before Breaking Down?

How much force, how much movement, how much carrying your child on your hip can you tolerate before your body starts letting you know it's breaking down in response to whatever it is that you're doing? Remember that the objective is to build a body you love to live in, not build a body that's constantly on the edge of getting hurt. The tolerance of your tissues refers to how much force they can take and still maintain themselves, and it plays a role in how your tissues feel, what they can do, and how resistant to future aches and injuries you are. To understand tissue tolerance, we should look to something called the 'zone of homeostasis'.

First put forth by Scott Dye in 1996, the zone of homeostasis is one of four zones that relate to your tissues and the forces being placed on them. Remember, forces come by way of movement, impact (such as someone knocking into you), the things you pick up and carry, whether weights in the gym or a dog who refuses to walk the rest of the way home, the body positions you assume, and even the clothes and shoes you wear. The zone of homeostasis is considered to be the range, or 'zone', within which your tissues and joints can accept a broad range of forces and maintain homeostasis of the tissue. Tissue homeostasis means that the complex physiological processes which are constantly happening at the cellular level are able to keep going, and your tissues just keep on keepin' on.

What the zone of homeostasis suggests is that you've got a particular range of forces that can be placed on your tissues that won't disrupt your tissues from maintaining their cellular processes that keep them healthy and functional. If you experience loading on your tissues that is outside of that zone, you increase the likelihood that you'll experience tissue issues (a.k.a. injuries), perhaps micro, or perhaps macro in nature.

Here's what Dye said about this in a research paper he published:

"A single loading event of sufficient magnitude or a series of repetitive loading events of a lesser magnitude can cause an injury, inducing a cascade of reparative biochemical processes which reflect a loss, at least temporarily, of normal tissue homeostasis."[20]

---

20   Dye, Scott F MD. (2005 July). The Pathophysiology of Patellofemoral Pain: A Tissue Homeostasis Perspective. *Clinical Orthopaedics and Related Research: July 2005 - Volume 436 - Issue - p 100-110* doi: 10.1097/01.blo.0000172303.74414.7d.

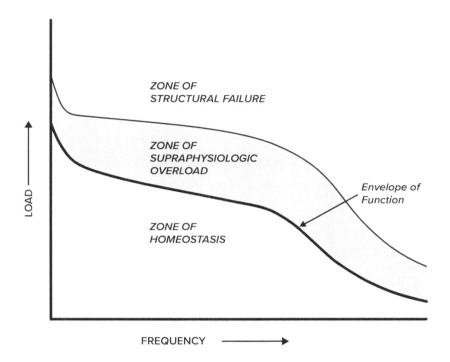

So you've got your zone of homeostasis, and at the very edge of it is what Dye called the 'envelope of function'. This is where you find the upper limit of the force and frequency of force your tissues can tolerate before homeostasis in your tissues gets disrupted. Not to give the answer too soon, but the zone of homeostasis and its upper limit signified by the envelope of function are where you'd ideally spend the majority of your time operating.

Once you pass your envelope of function, you move into what is called the 'zone of supraphysiologic overload'. It's in this zone where forces placed on your body are either too much and/or too frequent for you to respond to appropriately, but not so far past your tissues' capability that you'll sustain a structural failure like a fractured bone or ruptured ACL. Issues that arise here are more likely to be muscle strains, tendinopathy, inflammation that's disruptive but not overwhelming to your system, and a disruption of tissue homeostasis that could feel like stiff muscles and joints.

Dye uses the example of long-distance running (and the classic mistake of doing too much, too soon) to demonstrate the zone of supraphysiologic overload when the frequency is too high. Distance running is not a massive amount of load — it's just your bodyweight plus gravity meeting the pavement with each step you take — but it is a high frequency of loading, as you are doing it for a long period of time. Note that 'long' is relative here… 'long' for an off-the-couch runner might be three miles, while 'long' for an experienced endurance runner might be going straight from running five miles to running ten or more.

A common example of too much force is when someone doing resistance training exercises chooses weights that are too heavy for their current capacity but not so heavy they can't lift them at all. They grunt and push their way through the exercise, but their technique suffers and they struggle to complete the exercise. Whether too much force or too great a frequency of force, if you do more of it than your tissues can readily tolerate you'll be operating in your zone of supraphysiologic overload. Dye noted that there are "indicators that a given joint is being loaded beyond its envelope of function which would include pain, discomfort, functional instability, and the presence of effusion, warmth, and tenderness…"[21]

There are two issues that arise when you spend too much time in the zone of supraphysiologic overload, in addition to the reality that you might experience a painful sensation if you push beyond the envelope of function. First, if you consistently exert yourself with enough force or enough frequency of force that you're perpetually working in your zone of supraphysiologic overload, your tissues aren't getting a chance to fully recover from this overload. The resultant tissue imbalance can make it difficult to return to tissue homeostasis (which allows the tissues to heal and grow stronger). When normal tissue homeostasis becomes imbalanced, tissue function can become impaired, causing changes to how the tissue functions.

This can then cause your envelope of function to actually drop down and to the left, thereby making everyday activities difficult or painful when they were not previously. Anyone who has overdone it with a workout knows the sensation — just going down a flight of stairs the next day or sitting down on the toilet feels painful. In this case, over-

21   Dye, Scott F MD. (1996 April). The Knee as a Biologic Transmission With an Envelope of Function, *Clinical Orthopaedics and Related Research: April 1996 - Volume 325 - Issue - p 10-18*. Retrieved from https://journals.lww.com/clinorthop/Fulltext/1996/04000/The_Knee_as_a_Biologic_Transmission_With_an.3.aspx

doing the forces or frequency of forces to the tissues during your workout can make basic everyday activities more of a stressor on your tissues.

In addition, spending too much time in this zone can also trigger an increase in stimuli that your nerve endings detect and interpret as a painful sensation and report it up to your brain. The more those nerve receptors pick up potentially noxious stimuli, the more indication your brain gets that there might be a reason to create pain. As you might recall from the pain chapter, your brain can get more proficient at feeling pain because those nerves are being stimulated so frequently, which means an acute event can turn into a chronic tissue issue where pain then becomes more consistently present.

This is not to say you should never enter the zone of supraphysiologic overload, and in fact, one way to build more tissue tolerance is to thoughtfully and intentionally dip over into it. A well-constructed physical training program will do this, and I can't stress those words enough. *Well-constructed* means there are sound progressions of volume, frequency, and intensity in the program.

Lots of folks miss the mark on this one, thinking that constantly going hard and making the exercises very difficult equates to results. It does not. This is why it's so vitally important that you do not 'go big or go home' when taking up any sort of more active lifestyle or physical training program. Appropriate dosage and appropriate increase of the dosage wins out every time. In my Unbreakable Body workout program, folks are frequently surprised at how mild the progressions are in terms of volume, frequency, and intensity. That surprise comes about, I think, because it's just so common to hear that exercise has to push you to the limit and beyond in order to be effective. But that's just not the case.

Next, we move beyond the zone of supraphysiologic overload into the zone where macrostructural failure of your tissues, joints, or bones occurs. This is known as the zone of structural failure. Remember my ACL rupture from that climbing fall? That's a good example here: the sudden force of my bodyweight, plus gravity, plus momentum on the structures of my knee, and in the position it was in when I hit the ground, caused a macrostructural failure to the ligament, causing a rupture.

While it's obvious that staying out of this zone is ideal, it's not possible to guarantee that you'll never find yourself in a position where the forces on your tissues are far in excess of what they can tolerate. You might trip and fall, you might be in a car accident, you might run into another player during your recreational volleyball game. There is no way to avoid risk, especially if you want to live your life fully. But what you can do is increase what your tissues can tolerate in the zones below the zone of structural failure. The benefit of this is two-fold.

One, if you have greater tissue tolerance in the zones below structural failure, you have more and greater forces you can tolerate before you cross into zones where micro or macro structural damage can occur. And two, if you have greater tissue tolerance *and you do happen to sustain an injury*, you're likely to bounce back more quickly if you are starting from a place of strength. This is how you build resistance and resilience in your body.

Here are a few examples of what it looks like to increase your tissue tolerance:

If going for a run three days a week puts you past your envelope of function, start with fewer days per week of running. Or, start with walking most days of the week. By either doing a similar amount of force (running) but less frequently, or doing less force but more frequently (walking), and slowly increasing the amount or frequency, in time you'll find that going running three times a week no longer puts you past your envelope of function.

If doing the weightlifting workout as it's written requires you to lift weights that are beyond your envelope of function and in turn your body feels absolutely crushed in the days that follow the workout, start with using a lighter weight or doing fewer sets of the exercises in the workout. Build up your ability to tolerate that amount and frequency of force such that you come out of the workout feeling great and ready for more, rather than crushed beyond recognition. In time, your tissues will increase their tolerance and you'll be ready to go up in both weights and sets in your workout.

Increasing tissue tolerance is not just for achieving fitness gains or healing an injury. It's also for making you more capable in your life. I had a client once, a spunky lady in her 70s, who would hold household objects, such as cans of soup, in her hands with her arm out in front of her for increasing lengths of time. As she put it, "I wanted to see if I could and most people my age can't. And at first I couldn't do it for very long myself so I decided to see if I could get better at it." Right on, woman. Smart, too, because grip strength has been shown to have an inverse correlation with death risk, that is, the stronger your grip the less risk you have of dying.[22]

All too often, body care for aches, pains, and injuries is only done when you have an ache, a pain, or an injury. When there's no aches, pains, or injuries, body care drops off or is forgotten. But now that you know about the zones of tissue tolerance, what usefulness is it to be less active in your day?

What if, instead of treating body care as an emergency solution, you treated it as something you always need and that always benefits you? What if you took time in your day — not your workout time, not your yoga class time — but moments throughout the entire day and infused them with signals to tell your body how you want it to respond so that you fortify that zone of homeostasis?

Your day is already full of signals your body is responding to anyway, so you may as well join the conversation and

22   Leong, Darryl, MD et al. (2015) Prognostic value of grip strength: findings from the PURE study. The Lancet, 386 (9990) 266-273 Retrieved from https://www.thelancet.com/journals/lancet/article/PIIS0140-6736(14)62000-6/fulltext

curate those signals to support your Unbreakable body in the ways that you need. In doing so, body care stops being a band-aid for a problem and starts being the glue that holds you together.

"But just doing a little bit isn't *really* going to make an impact, so why bother?" Listen, humans usually aren't intrinsically good at intentionally doing a little bit consistently over time. It's why studies have repeatedly shown that the best way to save for retirement is to have your employer auto-draft a set amount of money each month before you even see your paycheck. It's also why studies show that the diet that works best is the one you can keep doing forever. It is no different for your body and your care of it. Little bits done consistently don't just work better: they radically change the way you navigate your experience of living in your body, especially when it comes to tending to aches and pains.

What I am asking you to consider is how you can make your life richer in signals that cultivate the responses you desire from your body. The simplest way to start curating the signals you send your body is to take something you already do and tack onto it a small action that signals to your body that there's something new you want it to respond to. That way you're not having to carve out a big block of time to do the signal-sending, but just adding it on to something you already do. This makes it much easier to ensure it gets done.

Now, I don't know what your schedule entails compared to mine, but chances are we have a few similar touchpoints in our days, like meal times. For instance, at breakfast, you might do a few repetitions of a slow, controlled, circle of your neck, exploring how it feels as you move it, noticing where it is noisy and crinkly. At lunch, you could do the toe-lift exercises I teach you in the book bonus while you sit and eat. At dinnertime, before you sit down to eat, you could do a few rotations of your wrists, slow and controlled, exploring how those tissues in your wrists and forearms that were bothering you a bit at the end of your work day are feeling now.

The benefits of enriching your life with body care signals are many.

First, a little bit of movement each day, over weeks and months, adds up. Five repetitions of a seemingly simple neck motion might seem like nothing to you, but it's not nothing to your body's tissues.

Second, when you have a few movements you do every day, you notice more quickly when something feels different, off, or worse. This awareness can help you do a form of triage where you can shift your attention and your actions, and prioritize tending to that area to help it respond more favorably once again, rather than having no awareness of the area until it's really screaming at you that your attention is needed.

Third, by intentionally including signals to your body to help it respond in the manner you desire, you assist in maintaining the health and function of your tissues. Remember, your body is always responding, and if you stop signaling to your body that maintenance and upkeep of those particular tissues is a priority, it will stop. This is one of the most common ways a person loses range of motion and strength in their body: they just stop using it.

Finally, enriching your life with body care signals automatically makes you more aware and in tune to how you move, how you don't move, what you're doing with your body, how you're sitting, the way you lean on one leg more than the other, and so on. By tuning in more, you get to know yourself better. You might not have much time in your day, but what could you do with the time you do have?

Before we move on, we need to fill in the last zone on this four-zone model. This last zone is the zone where your tissues have not experienced enough load in order to maintain homeostasis, and it's called the zone of subphysiologic underload. Recall that tissue structure and the cellular activity within the tissues are heavily influenced by forces being placed on the tissue. In times when there's not enough force placed on the tissue to do those things appropriately (such as prolonged bed rest, inactivity, de-training, and immobilization) this can create muscle atrophy, a loss of bone density, and a reduction in the processes which maintain tissue homeostasis. By moving your body regularly and exposing it to forces consistently, you'll make your zone of subphysiologic underload a non-issue.

Now, lest you think that there's a perfect way to know what zone you're operating in, Dye noted in his paper that these zones are likely not as clearly defined as they look to be when placed on a graph. With the exception of loads that trigger structural failure — where there's a fairly clear line between 'failure' and 'not failure' of the tissue — the rest of the zones more likely blend together, rather than there being distinct demarcations between one to the next. In addition, the zones will probably vary depending on which tissue is being considered — for example, when I fell and ruptured my ACL, neither my leg bone nor my muscles experienced structural failure, but my ligament did. Third, these zones are not fixed, meaning they can and will change over time, moving more up and to the right or down and to the left, based on your actions or inactions. Fourth, because your body is a complex organization of interconnected systems, it's likely that the zones will fluctuate based on things beyond the realm of physical training, or the lack thereof. Things like your total stress load, sleep quality, diet, health status, and more will also influence your zones of tissue tolerance.

This is why it pays to be tapped into your Explorer's Mindset so that you can be perpetually exploring, experimenting, and curating information to aid you as you make decisions that build your tissue tolerance and become Unbreakable. If you overdid it in your workouts last week, or in your yardwork last weekend, it's not the end of the world. Simply use that information to take note and adjust course for next time.

My Body Boke Down. Now What?

After an injury, your zones of tissue tolerance around the injury site (and perhaps in additional areas depending on the nature of the injury), are likely to shift down and to the left, limiting the movements you can do or the positions you can assume.

Anyone who has sprained an ankle knows this sensation — putting your full bodyweight on the ankle right after the injury often feels impossible, even though you could bear all that weight on the ankle without issue in the moments before the injury. When tissues exceed their envelope of function and sustain mild stress and strain, or more significant structural failure, their ability to tolerate force will be reduced until you can rebuild that higher tolerance. In the case of structural failure, a period of immobilization while the tissue regains a base level of tolerance is usually necessary. If you've broken a bone, you'll probably be put into a cast, and if you've torn a ligament, tendon, or muscle, you'll likely be encouraged to avoid putting any force on that area for a period of time. But that doesn't mean you have to treat the other tissues outside of the injured area the same way. Provided you're staying out of painful positions, and you're not breaking any guidelines given to you by your doc (if you met with one), you can re-start the process of fortifying your tissue tolerance in all the rest of your tissues of your body.

Whether you're working on restoring after a big injury

or you're working on a milder strain or sprain type of issue, you can start sending signals to your tissues by slowly and consistently exposing them to movement or exercise that challenges those particular tissues and gradually increasing in amount, frequency, and intensity over time. Building tissue tolerance after an injury is a similar protocol to how you build your tissue tolerance for fitness and performance, it really is two sides of the same coin. Gradually increase the amount of forces and frequency of forces that your tissues face and over time your tissues will become more tolerant of those forces. It's true whether you're trying to build tolerance to be able to stand with full bodyweight on your ankle again, or if you're trying to build tolerance to lift very heavy weights in the gym.

This is what a clinician will do when they construct a rehab program for you, and while I strongly recommend you work with a professional when healing an injury, you also don't have to limit your rehab to the time you spend with them or the few minutes it takes to do your homework exercises. In fact, knowing that low-level, gentle, movements that involve the injured tissues at a level of force that is tolerable for the current state of your tissues is an effective way to assist in rehabilitation and to help you be more proactive after an injury.

It's very motivating after an injury to know that the power is in your hands, simply by sending signals through various forces so your tissues can organize and adapt themselves to become more tolerant of that force in the future. When you know that you lead the charge on this healing journey, and that anyone who you bring on to help — like a doctor or clinician — is there to *assist* you, not take over your role as the leader, you experience a level of confidence that will serve as the driving force for you do the work to heal the injury.

Examples of simple movements that impart forces into tissues include moving the affected area through as much range of motion as you can without pain: flexing, extending, or rotating the affected joint, contracting the muscles of the affected area isometrically, this just means 'without movement' (If you contract your leg muscles right now by stiffening them without moving any part of your leg while you sit or lay down, that's an isometric contraction.)

With all of the motions and muscle contractions you're doing, the injured tissues will respond to those signals and increase their tolerance for the forces you're placing on them. In due time, you'll be able to bear your full body weight on the injured area or start using whatever part of your body that was injured at max capacity once again. And of course, you can keep going from there, building your tissue tolerance so you can handle even more than you could originally..

And if you experience an injury and would really like to take action to rebuild your tissue tolerance, but are worried that you'll do something that makes things worse, here are three suggestions:

1) Ask your clinician (if you're working with one) as many questions as you can about what you can do, how much you can do, and if there is anything you should be aware of regarding the injury and the healing process. They have knowledge and expertise that you might not have, and their job is to share that with you so that you can put it to use as you make choices for your body.

2) Build trust in yourself that you won't make things worse by practicing using the minimum effective dose. Chances are, if you don't have strong trust in yourself about your body, there's a reason for it. It may be a good reason, or it may be a reason that was once good but has outlived its usefulness. You can use your Explorer's Mindset to dig into the reasoning behind it, but in terms of actions you can take, the minimum effective dose is a useful one. Here's how it works: the minimum effective dose of something is the lowest dose that provides a beneficial response. (There is also a maximum effective dose, and you can certainly work up to finding that, but if you struggle to trust that you won't overdo it, you might need some practice before you get there.)

To find your minimum effective dose, all you need to do is start with one repetition of whatever movement or muscle contraction you want to make. Just one! Then see how you feel — allow your body to inform you of whether it tolerated that one repetition or not. After that, you can try two repetitions, and repeat this process until you find an amount of movement that feels good (which will likely be far less than you think you "should" be able to do and which does not leave you feeling like you're in a deficit of fatigue, soreness, weakness, or anything else.

You should feel just plain good after doing your minimum effective dose. Then work with that amount of repetitions for a period of time and pay attention to how your body responds. After a time, which might be a few days, or a week or more depending on where you are starting from, add another repetition or two. Then watch how your body responds. Continue on in this manner staying within that realm of volume of work which your body responds favorably to.

Remember, the Signal/Response Principle is always working, so these small doses of movement are still creating responses in your body. Now, you might want to do more than the minimum effective dose, hoping to make faster progress. But if you're trying to develop trust in yourself that you won't make the injury worse, remember that building that trust is the point here, not being the fastest at recovery. Recovery will happen, and it won't take forever. Build that level of trust and respect for what your body is communicating to you.

3) Even if you don't trust yourself yet, remember that

your brain is wired for keeping you safe and alive. In the pain chapter we talked about how your brain and the rest of your nervous system are always alert and looking out for possible threats. Your brain and nervous system are still doing that even as you heal. They're like a buddy who is looking out for you, so let yourself operate knowing that they'll let you know if you're heading towards a possible threat.

Through experimenting, you'll be able to find the right ratio of the signals you're choosing to send to aid your tissues in healing from their ache or injury, and get yourself on the path of "calming stuff down and building stuff up."

But What About Resting It?

Rest was a cornerstone of the acronym RICE (which stands for Rest, Ice, Compression, and Elevation), which was used for a very long time as the standard method for treating injuries. Unfortunately, the evidence doesn't support this approach, and even the creator of the RICE acronym put out a statement retracting his support for the method, not only because aspects of RICE do not seem to work, but they have shown to actually delay healing.

RICE was put forth by Dr. Gabe Mirkin in his 1978 book, *The Sports Medicine Book*,[23] and one line in his retrac-

---

23 Mirkin G. & Hoffman M. (1978) *The Sports Medicine Book*. Boston, Massachusetts, USA: Little, Brown &Co

tion statement sums things up: "Both ice and complete rest may delay healing instead of helping." Rest ensures that no forces are placed on the tissue that would surpass the tissue's current zone of homeostasis, but rest also means no forces are placed on the tissue that *meet* the tissue's current zone of homeostasis. Thus, there are no signals to tell your tissue how you want it to respond. And as you now know, force is paramount for telling tissues how they should adapt and respond, and the more particular the force, the more particular the response of increased tissue tolerance.

In addition to sending forces that guide your tissue to heal and build its tolerance, you need inflammation as part of the healing process. Inflammation is your immune system's response to injured tissue and when tissue damage has occurred, cells called macrophages rush to the area and release a hormone called IGF-1, which helps injured tissues to heal. Ice diminishes the release of IGF-1, thereby slowing the healing process.

Dr. Mirkin goes on to say that "anything that reduces inflammation also delays healing. Thus, healing is delayed by cortisone-type drugs, almost all pain-relief medicines, immune suppressants that are often used to treat arthritis, applying cold packs or ice, and anything else that blocks the immune response to healing."[24] And so, aside from certain

---

24   Mirkin, G. (2015 September 16). Why Ice Delays Recovery [Blog post]. Retrieved from https://www.drmirkin.com/fitness/why-ice-delays-recovery.html

'runaway' inflammatory conditions, where inflammation has gotten out of control and needs management, it's important to allow the inflammatory process to occur. Think of 'rest' as a signal to your tissues just as you think of movement as a signal to them. Is the response your body will make to 'rest' the kind of response you want? Answer that in each scenario and you'll have your answer as to "should I rest this part of my body?"

Activities you can do to increase your tissue tolerance can be broad, where you're simply focusing on moving in a general way and doing a little bit more next time than you did this time. Or, they can be highly specific, focusing on moving a particular joint and contracting a particular muscle at a particular angle at a particular intensity for a particular amount of time. In the case of an ankle sprain injury, build your tissues up so they tolerate more forces in all of the particular positions in which your ankle may find itself in the future (highly specific), and you would want to build their ability to tolerate general movement, such as when going out for your walk and aiming to go five minutes longer this week than last before your ankle got tired (broad and more general). Recall that at the cellular level, your tissues will reorganize and orient themselves along the lines of tension that the force imparts, which in turn makes stronger, better, tissues.

My Body Is Just Achy, Not Broken Down. What About That?

"I don't think I'm injured, but my back doesn't feel good." That's how one client described it when we were talking about what they were feeling in their body. Those aches that aren't severe enough to stop you in your tracks but that you're aware of and that don't feel good are probably the most common things you'll come across when taking care of your body ecosystem.

They're also most likely to be the body responses that make you feel the worst about living in your body — they rack up over the years, make you feel old and tired, and unlike tripping and spraining an ankle, they often seem to show up without you having done something to cause them. What in the world do we do about those?

When you move your body, whether to stand, sit, reach for something, exercise, run, hug someone, or anything else, your body responds in a multitude of ways. These responses happen lightning fast, as soon as you initiate motion (whether consciously or unconsciously), including coordinating muscle contractions, moving one or many joints in a coordinated fashion, bracing some parts of you, allowing motion to other parts, breathing in a particular manner, and dispersing forces across a few or many tissues of your body. The tissues and joints that you're dispersing forces across are each well-suited for particular duties, though they can also be put to use in ways they're not quite as well suited for.

For example: imagine you're reaching for an object above your head, perhaps a bowl on the top shelf of your kitchen cabinets. Here's a glimpse into what's happening biomechanically when you raise your arm up. Your upper arm bone (the humerus) will move within the main joint of your shoulder (the glenohumeral joint). Your shoulder blade (called the scapula) will also move along your ribcage in conjunction with your arm raising up. Attached to all of these bones are soft tissues — muscles, tendons, ligaments, joint capsule tissues, fascia, and skin — all of which will contract and move as you reach your arm upward. Additionally, your brain is determining where your body is in space and how much muscle contraction it must make for each tissue involved in the process of reaching, not to mention keeping you balanced so you don't fall over while you reach. Simple movement is truly quite a feat!

But what if your body can't do one of those things? What if your arm and shoulder joint don't seem to be able to move very much? What if your muscles don't have the strength to raise your arm high enough? What if your balance has diminished the last few years and you feel wobbly when you reach? What if you don't know what it is that your body can't do, all you know is that reaching doesn't feel good? Are you simply out of luck?

Thankfully, if you need to move your body, your brain and body will adapt to the current circumstances and you'll select a strategy to accomplish the task at hand. And most times, you'll do this without even realizing you're doing it. You might shrug your upper back, shoulder, and neck muscles up into your ear to help lift your arm up. You might twist your body to make the reaching arm move closer to the thing you're reaching for. You might make all sorts of adjustments to make it so your body can do the thing you're asking it to do with the things it's got available for the job. Folks tend to call these adjustments 'compensations'. I believe a better word for them is 'accommodations'.

Consider this: when you accommodate someone, you're providing something for them, helping them out, or adapting something to make it suitable for them — letting them stay in your spare bedroom, lending them money, or switching seats with them at the big group dinner because they're left-handed (as left-handers know, the left end seat is the ideal seat — you don't get your elbow smashed and bashed when sitting to the right of a right-hander who is free-wheeling their elbow around).

Conversely, the word 'compensating' tends to provoke a sense of doing one thing because you don't have enough of something else. The old trope of the guy who buys the flashy sports car to cover for some supposed insecurity is a good example. Now, whether you buy a sports car because you like them or because you're compensating for something, it doesn't matter to me. But when it comes to your body, try on the idea of your body *accommodating* you, rather than *compensating* for you. Your nervous system — and thus, your body — is always accommodating you. And accommodations aren't wrong or bad, but they do create effects, or responses.

Bodies will do whatever you ask of them with whatever means they have to do it. If you over-rely on some tissues compared to others, or use tissues in a way they're not entirely well-suited for, then that achy back and stiff shoulder might merely be your body trying to do what you want it to and letting you know they're not exactly suited for that job. Instead of feeling like this is just to be expected as you get older, consider that perhaps the solution is to learn how to move your tissues and joints in new ways so you can disperse forces more effectively and efficiently across them so that each joint and tissue can do its job effectively, efficiently, and with ease. This is an important result you can get from exercise that is so often overlooked because exercise is often seen as something you do to change your body composition or to get strong for a sport or activity you enjoy. And there's nothing wrong with using exercise as a way to achieve either of those things, but at a fundamental level, exercise is capable of helping you become a better mover of your body. And when you become a better mover of your body and all its parts, you become more capable of doing the workouts and sports you love, thereby removing hurdles from your path.

To become a better mover and have fewer body accommodations that create little aches and pains along the way, simply give your body more options to choose from. Give it more accommodations that can work for you without sending your tissues into the land of Achesville. You already know about building tissue tolerance, next it's time to introduce you to the Six Pillars of an Unbreakable body. Tissue tolerance is the 'what' to focus on, the Six Pillars are the 'where' to focus on. Before we head into that, a final reminder as we leave this chapter on aches and injuries: every ache and injury — no matter how long it takes to figure it out and resolve it — is a lesson. A lesson in discovering an area of opportunity you previously may not have known about. A lesson in improving your order of prioritization for body care. A lesson in honing your confidence that while external factors will happen to you, you're in charge of what comes next.

This is a cornerstone of becoming Unbreakable — taking aches, tweaks, and injuries that occur and using them to get stronger and better than you were before. There is always something to learn from even the most annoying of injuries, not the least of which is, "how can I make myself less susceptible to this injury in the future?" The exploration, data collection, experimentation, and curation of signals that help you achieve the responses you desire truly never ends.

PART FOUR:

Building Your Unbreakable Body

CHAPTER 14:

Introducing the Six Pillars

At the start of this book, I told you about Ruth and Steve, and how they became Unbreakable. They proved wrong the myth that you can reach 'too late' while you're still alive and they become experts in the care of their bodies because they refused to believe that it could be 'too complicated' for them.

Both also maintained steady forward momentum by building a base of physical capacity and fitness that supported their every move. This base is made up of the Six Pillars of an Unbreakable body. These six areas of the body are a dynamic framework that flow with you from beginning to end of the journey you're on in this lifetime, from building your body up to a level that works well for you, to sustaining your body as you take on more specific goals and endeavors, to maintaining your body as you hit the age everyone tells you is the age your body will fall apart on you. The Six Pillars are not a rigid to-do list to accomplish, but rather, they give you areas to focus on while also ensuring you can always tailor your efforts to exactly what your body needs.

Before we dive into what the Six Pillars are and how you work with them in your body, I want to illustrate the impact of tending to them by sharing the story of my client, Joe. When we met, Joe had the standard view of exercise and body care — that is, you do exercise to achieve an end goal, like losing weight, or to fix a problem, like when he had shoulder surgery and they sent him to physical therapy for a few months afterward to regain his strength. And while you can use exercise and body care activities for these things, Joe didn't have the whole picture of how exercise and body care activities can be such powerful tools for helping him build a body he loved to live in.

Thus far, Joe's efforts to thwart the aches and pains that crept up in his body had been feeling like a game of whack-a-mole. If you're not familiar with that old arcade game, you hold a soft club and try to whack a mechanical mole that pops out of various holes with maddening randomness. You really never make progress in this game — the mole is too fast — so you just end up in a violent frenzy while people watching you play this silly game stand around laughing. While that makes for a fun time at an arcade, it's not a fun time if that's how you're feeling in your body.

For Joe, the game of bodily whack-a-mole looked like this: first, he had hip pain that had been bothering him and so he tried over-the-counter pain-relief medicine. But it quickly became apparent that the medicine only really worked for a short time and he knew he couldn't just keep popping pills forever.

Next, he tried a series of stretches that he found online when he searched the internet for information on 'hip pain'. He did the stretches consistently for a month and his hip pain improved marginally, but he wanted more measurable progress, so his next idea was to go for monthly massages in addition to doing the hip stretches. The massages definitely gave him some relief from the hip pain, and after a few months of massages and stretching, he felt well enough to stop both.

However, it wasn't long before he started feeling twinges on the outer edge of his knee. His doctor said nothing was structurally wrong and prescribed him stretches to do, so Joe got back to work doing those. Unlike the last series of stretches though, these didn't seem to do anything for him. He then purchased a knee brace to see if that would help at all and wore it for any activities that he did during his non-work time, like when he went out to do yard work and when he and the kids went out on bike rides. The brace helped him forget about his knee while he was doing these activities, and that was a big win in his book. However, when he wasn't wearing the brace, he still felt the twinges on the outer edge of his knee. It was around that time that Joe and I met.

Whacking at problems when they arise and taking actions that manage the symptom rather than the root cause are both a form of symptom-focused action, not one that considers the ecosystem as a whole. There's a time and place for symptom-focused action, to be sure. For instance, if you break your arm, you will most certainly want to put a cast on the broken bone so it can heal without being jostled as you move about your day. But there's a common mistake in exercise and body care, which is to narrow the scope of problem-solving to the tiniest view, only considering the area where the pain, weakness, or issue has arisen, and never broadening the scope to include the rest of the ecosystem you're living in, or how everything in the ecosystem is interacting.

This frenzied symptom-whacking is what happens when an ecosystem is managed as if it's not one. "What is the one exercise I need to be doing to make my back strong?" "What is the one thing I need to do to get this pain to subside?" "Which treatment/brace/workout program will get rid of this issue now?" There's no answer to those questions, because they're the wrong questions.

Ecosystems (including your body) by their very nature are full of interdependent parts and subsystems that influence each other. When you try to single out solutions, you oversimplify the problem by an order of magnitude. The singular solutions Joe had been trying worked for a bit, but they weren't adding up to a whole body that felt progressively better over time, and they certainly weren't helping him feel Unbreakable. I introduced Joe to the Six Pillars of an Unbreakable body, and through our workouts together, Joe began to experience what it's like to take care of his body as a complete ecosystem.

As he built his Six Pillars, he experienced what it feels like to accumulate steady progress and a solid base of physical capacity, and as he resolved his aches and pains, he was able to start tackling the physical fitness goals he was most excited by without the starts and stops he'd experienced in the past when he was dealing with recurring aches and pains. He stopped feeling like he was playing whack-a-mole with his body, which gave him back both the mental and physical energy that he'd previously been spending on reacting to the various issues that would pop up.

Knowing how to use the Six Pillars framework helped him build more confidence in his abilities to take care of his body, so that he could do whatever he liked with it. This meant he could say 'yes' more often to activities life presented him with — from coaching soccer for his kids' team to crawling into the crawl space of his house to get storage items out (something that had been a struggle in the past, and which always ended up in a tweaky back or shoulder).

As he brought his unique vision of what it means to be

Unbreakable to life, he also learned how to tune in, take care, and listen to his body at a level that he'd not experienced before. And so Joe, who'd been trying his best to deal with his body prior to building his Six Pillars, joined Ruth and Steve in creating a body he loved to live in.

What are the Six Pillars?

The Six Pillars of an Unbreakable body are a framework I developed that take all this complex material and organize it into an easy-to-use tool for tending to your body ecosystem in a more holistic way. You certainly could go about memorizing all of the muscles of the body, what their actions are, and the multitude of things that influence them, plus all of the other systems and processes that your marvelous body undertakes every day, and if you've got that much time and are that interested in the rabbit hole of exercise science, by all means do that. But whether you want to dive down rabbit holes or you really don't have the interest or time for that much research, the Six Pillars framework will help you get better results for yourself.

For my clients, having a framework helps them achieve the results they want, and it helps them take the reins on their own physical training and body care. The Six Pillars guide your attention to key areas of your body that — when they have enough of what they need — create a solid base upon which you can layer everything else.

The Six Pillars are simple to work with, and they can be

layered into anything you do — daily life, sports you take on, new activities you pursue — to help ensure you cover your bases in your exercise and body care. Learning how to work with the Six Pillars provides you a lifetime of confidence in yourself as the caretaker of your Unbreakable body because you become an expert in adapting your physical training and lifestyle to suit you and your body's needs. It's why the Six Pillars framework is not an on/off thing where either you're 'doing the program' or you're not. You *can* treat it like a diet where you're 'on' or you're 'off' but it's far more effective, impactful, and low stress, when you begin to include the Six Pillars framework as something you can put to work for you one way or another for the rest of your life.

Listing them from the ground up, the Six Pillars are: Strong Feet, Mobile Hips, Strong Glutes, Strong Torso, Mobile Shoulders, and Strong Posture. We are going to go over them in greater detail in a different order though, thanks to how the information builds on itself.

Pillar #1: Strong Torso

The first Pillar to discuss is a Strong Torso. While there was a long history of infomercials focusing on building "abs of steel", building a strong torso isn't about that at all. In fact, making your torso into something akin to a piece of metal that doesn't bend or break is actually the opposite of what you're after here. Your torso needs to be able to move and flow, allowing for things like appropriate inhalation and exhalation as you breathe, it needs to house your internal organs, and to support you through the wide array of positions needed to navigate life with ease.

If you've ever experienced pain in your back, or developed a muscle strain in your abdomen or rib cage, or who felt like you don't have the ability to brace your body to pick up things without injury, you know that having a strong torso is paramount. But in order to get a strong torso, we first need to clarify what we mean by *strong* and *torso*.

First, what is included when I say *torso*? The torso is not just the "abs" or "core" muscles. When we build a strong torso, we're focused on the diaphragm muscle, the abdominal muscles, the pelvic floor muscles (which are also called the 'pelvic diaphragm', and support your torso from below), the muscles that lie between each rib of your ribcage, your chest muscles, as well as accessory breathing muscles like the muscles of your neck, and the ribcage itself. When we think about the strong torso, we're thinking about everything from the neck to bottom of the pelvis.

Next, what is meant by *strength*? Strength can be demonstrated in a multitude of ways, but building a strong torso for an Unbreakable human is, first and foremost, about being able to find and maintain a stacked position of the skeletal structures and torso muscles, so that you can do three very important actions that you'll need to call on every single day. They are: breathing, moving, and managing the internal pressures necessary to withstand external forces.

We'll talk more about breathing and moving in just a moment, but you might be thinking that you're not familiar with this concept of internal pressure management. But in fact, you've experienced it every day of your life. You have a level of pressure inside of your torso which needs to be at least as strong as the external pressure being exerted on your body, whether the external pressure is simply the everyday nature of gravity pressing on you, or it is something more strenuous or complex, like coordinating the movement of getting into and out of a car, or picking up something heavy.

This internal pressure is managed by your body through muscle contractions so that the internal pressure of your torso changes to meet the external pressures without breaking down under them. A few notable examples of pressure changes are: using the toilet, doing resistance training, and sneezing. When the internal pressure is at least as strong as the external pressure, your torso is able to maintain its strength and integrity. When it's not, things like hernias, pelvic floor prolapse, urination during activity, and muscle strains can occur.

It's much easier to maintain internal pressure when you've got a good stacked position of your skeleton, and when you have muscular strength that can maintain that stack as you move. To picture this stacked position of your skeletal structures, imagine three jars stacked on top of each other, a small one on top, a big one in the middle, and a medium one down at the bottom. The small top jar represents your head, the middle one represents your ribcage, and the bottom one represents your pelvis.

Each of these three things —- your head, ribcage, and pelvis — are chambers that are made up of your bones and muscles, tendons, ligaments, and other soft tissues. Your head chamber is separated from your ribcage chamber by the vocal folds in your throat. Your ribcage and pelvic chambers are separated by your diaphragm. And as mentioned earlier, your pelvic chamber is supported by your pelvic floor muscles at the bottom.

When your body structures are stacked, it will look similar to how the jars look when you stack them up. That is, the top and bottom of each chamber are in alignment with each other (you don't have the top of the jar pointing one way and the bottom of that jar pointing another), and the bottom of one chamber faces the top of the next one (as opposed to having the jars all tipped in different directions and thus creating angles between the bottom of one and the top of another).

The jars are supported and stacked by "trunk muscles that act as one continuous functional unit, providing the core support for pressure regulation that allows the individual to multi-task, enabling 'walking, talking, and chewing gum' to occur simultaneously and effortlessly. In addition, the functions of the internal organs are supported by these pressures as well, especially the lungs, heart, vascular structures, gastrointestinal system and lymphatic systems."[25]

In addition to maintaining a stacked position to manage internal pressure effectively, having a stacked position of your three chambers also helps you to breathe effectively and efficiently. To explore breathing, we need to modify our three jars example now. Your three chambers do something really important which inanimate jars could never do, and that's oscillate, or shift, between compression and expansion.

As you inhale, all three of your chambers should expand. Yes, even your pelvis and head chambers move when you breathe, you just aren't as likely to feel or notice it. Then as you exhale, all three chambers should compress. And just as your nervous system needs to be able to oscillate between the two branches of the autonomic nervous system — rather than getting 'stuck' in one branch — these chambers of your body also need to be able to oscillate so that you can breathe and function well. We don't want them getting 'stuck' in expansion or compression.

You might be wondering how it's possible to get stuck in one or the other if at this very moment you are inhaling and exhaling, and thus, expanding and contracting. Your body will always accommodate you and find a way to get air in and move it back out however it can with whatever it has

25   Massery, M.,(2005). Musculoskeletal and neuromuscular interventions: a physical approach to cystic fibrosis. *Journal of the Royal Society of Medicine.* Supplement No 45, Volume 98, 55-62. Retrieved from http://www.masserypt.com/wp-content/uploads/2016/02/Massery-RSM-article.vol-98-sup-45p.55-662005.pdf

available for the job. But what is available might not be the things that are most well-suited for the job of breathing.

For example, if you lose the ability to fully expand your ribcage in all directions, your body might start using your neck and shoulders to lift the ribcage so air can go into your lungs. This works, but it's not ideal for the long-term as those muscles are not built to be the main respiratory muscles. You're getting air in, but not because your ribcage chamber is oscillating efficiently between expansion and contraction.

Efficient respiration means that the structures that normally coordinate breathing move into the right place at the right time so they can do the right thing. Ideally, your ribcage is able to expand adequately in all directions, front, sides, and back. You'd also like it to be able to compress all the way as you exhale, which the abdominals assist with, so that the diaphragm can be in an optimal position for the next breath you take. In addition to that, you'd like your pelvic floor to be able to descend downward and in harmony with your diaphragm up in your ribcage as you inhale, and then have it ascend again as you exhale.

When you are breathing quietly at rest, you'd like your neck, face, and upper shoulders to *not* be involved in creating muscular tension to lift the body upward in order to get air in — they should be able to remain quiet and at ease. And you'd like to be able to tolerate space between each breath, that is, you can complete the exhale and pause for a few seconds, without needing to inhale right away. It's all too common to think "I've done breathing exercises before, I already breathe correctly." You might. But you also might be quite surprised by what you find when you explore optimal respiratory mechanics, and how you breathe.

Because 'breathing training' has been commodified like so many things in fitness, there are a lot of breathing methods out there but as physical therapist, Dr. Anderson put it, "those are the 'what', but they often are not the 'how.' Interestingly, once you sort out breathing, torso strength comes more easily. As Dr. Anderson puts it, "Abs are for breathing performance, not core strength. Once you sort out breathing performance, core strength can naturally follow." You'll gain far more fitness and capability in building a strong torso simply by learning to breathe efficiently than you will from doing crunches.

Losing the stacked position of your three chambers can make it more difficult for those chambers to do all of these things effectively. And it goes in reverse as well: if you lose the ability to compress and expand well, it's going to be harder to find a stacked position with your three chambers. An interesting side effect of finding and maintaining the stacked position of these three chambers is that it can influence your nervous system's ability to oscillate between the sympathetic and parasympathetic branches. Back when I first introduced you to your nervous system, I mentioned something called the sympathetic ganglia that lies at the back of your ribcage. It should go from being compressed as you inhale to decompressed as you exhale, and this can inform your nervous system about whether it should ramp up into the sympathetic nervous system or restore the parasympathetic state. If you do not have efficient respiratory mechanics, the compression and decompression of your sympathetic ganglia can be impacted, which then leads your nervous system to stay more ramped up in the sympathetic nervous system response. A strong torso means a strong stack, which means a nice oscillation between expansion and compression, which means more efficient respiration, which means a nice oscillation between the branches of the autonomic nervous system.

As I mentioned earlier, finding and maintaining a stacked position of your three chambers also helps you move better. Movement requires that you generate force in your limbs to walk, push, pull, go up stairs, sit down in a chair, get up from the chair, twist, bend, or play a sport. It also requires that you coordinate the motion of your joints, as well as manage the varying changes to muscle tensions and muscle lengths required for you to move your joints, so that you can move as a functional unit that can accomplish the task at hand. Whether that task is picking up your child, carrying groceries in from the car, or going on an epic mountain bike ride on difficult terrain, being able to maintain a stacked position of the three chambers makes everything else you do more effective.

Think of it like this: when you move you are directing force towards something or away from something. In the case of carrying groceries in from the car, you want to be able to be weighed down by however many bags you've got and still be able to travel forward into the house. This requires that you direct force into holding the bags up while also pushing the ground away from you with each step you take.

To do this effectively, you want to be able to manage as much force as is necessary in each of those directions, holding up and pushing away. When you have a strong stacked position, you're able to drive energy to both, as there is no place else for that energy to go but to the task at hand. If you aren't able to maintain a strong stack, you'll inevitably leak energy as your body has to divert some of it to manage your torso position in addition to managing the motion you're doing. Finding a good stacked position of your torso helps you to close the windows, so to speak, so that there's no more drafty spaces and all your energy is directed to where you want it to go. By building the capacity of the muscles of your torso to manage the stacked position, you become more capable of supporting and stabilizing your skeleton as you move through all the positions of daily life.

The strength in a strong torso comes first from putting the body into a stacked position, then using a respiratory strategy that teaches the body to breathe efficiently and effectively in that position, and finally building the muscles to support the structures in maintaining the stacked position throughout each movement you want to do in life. Then you can layer on all of the sports and fitness training you could ever want and feel confident that you've built a strong base of structure and function that will be there for you when you go to lift heavy weights, or swing a softball bat, or carry your child on your hip as you go about your day. And on top of that, you build the ability of those muscles to work well for you when you want to do traditional abdominal or 'core' exercises, too. Whether you just want to get around the house without pain, or if you want to do heavy workouts, or if you want to go on adventures outdoors, you'll be able to train for all of it better and with greater effect when you've got your Strong Torso Pillar built up.

Here's an activity you can do to start finding the stacked position of a strong torso, and to incorporate efficient respiration. A demonstration of this activity and others are found on the book bonus web page: www.theunbreakablebody.com/book-bonus/ You'll want to either do this activity in shoes or barefoot, not in socks (you'll see why in a moment). You'll also want a prop that will be used to hold between your thighs, such as a pillow folded in half, or two towels rolled up into each other to form a cylinder. You want it to be about 4-6 inches in diameter.

- Find a place in your home where you can lie on the floor next to a wall. If you cannot get on the ground, you can also do this in bed, and where I use the wall in this activity, you'll use the headboard or wall that is by your bed. You might need to add some support with pillows behind your head, especially if your neck has to crane backwards to get your head to the floor.

- Lie on your back with your feet on the wall at a height where your ankles, knees, and hips are at right angles.

- Place the prop you selected between your thighs, and hold it there by squeezing your legs together gently.

- Bring your attention to your feet now, and make sure they are pointing straight up to the ceiling. Then start to feel how your feet are contacting the wall, specifically in three important areas: the ball joint of your big toe, the ball joint of your little toe, and your heel. Make those three points of contact connect firmly with the wall.

- Quietly inhale through your nose and as you exhale fully through your mouth, open your mouth and gently blow the air out, taking as long as you can to complete the exhale. . As you exhale, imagine that you're pulling your heels down the wall but instead of actually letting them slide down the wall, keep them in position. This is why you don't want to wear socks for this — they are too slippery and no matter how hard you keep contact with the bottom of your feet into the wall, your feet will still slide. We want zero sliding of the feet.

- Using that pulling down the wall motion of your heels (but remember, don't actually let them move!), curl the back of your pelvis up off the ground a few inches and allow your hips to raise up a few inches off the ground. Now, bring your attention to your hamstrings on the backs of your thighs. We want them to flex as you do this, so if they feel relaxed, try to increase the intensity of the pulling down of your heels motion. Note: if you've done the glute bridge exercise where you push your hips as high as you can, *this is not that*. This activity asks that instead of thrusting your hips up, you curl them up. Think of your pelvis as a bowl of soup, tuck your pelvis towards you, similarly to how you'd actually tip a soup bowl if you were to lift it up and sip directly from it.

- You'll hold these muscle contractions and focus points as you do the rest of the activity, so let's review them once more before moving on: the soles of your feet are connecting firmly with the wall through those three points of contact, your legs are lightly squeezing the prop between your legs, and your pelvis is holding a curled position as the hamstring muscles on the backs of your legs contract in response to the acting-as-if-pulling down motion of your heels.

- Maintaining those things, continue inhaling through your nose and exhaling through your mouth, and take your right arm and reach it up to the ceiling. Keep your back and head on the floor. The reaching should only come from your arm reaching from your shoulder joint, not from curling your body up or lifting your head. On your next exhale, reach your arm even further towards the ceiling, really reach! Aim to reach for a spot on the ceiling just over the midline of your body.

- Inhale and exhale again as you continue with and enhance all of the muscle contractions and focus points you're currently doing: your feet firmly contacting the wall, your legs squeezing the prop between the thighs, your heels acting-as-if-pulling down the wall and how that makes the backs of your legs contract, and the reach of your right arm from your shoulder.

- There are some other muscle contractions you might feel, too. You might feel your ribcage dropping down further into your body as you exhale; if so, wonderful! You might feel your abdominal muscles working, and while you don't need them to do a "crunch" move, they are likely to flex as you do this. You might feel a shaking sensation in your legs — that is common and often a sign that the muscles are working at a capacity or in a position that they're not as accustomed to and it may diminish as you do the activity more regularly.

You might feel your neck or face muscles tensing up. If so, these are respiratory accessory muscles and aren't made to be primary breathing muscles, so try and quiet them down. You might notice that you can't exhale for very long at first, but that's OK, because we'd like your primary breathing muscles — your diaphragm and your abdominal muscles — to get better at doing their job, and the only way they can is through practice.

And finally, you might feel your quadriceps muscles

on the tops of your thighs working. If so, they may be trying to help do the motion you're asking of your body because your body doesn't yet have another way of doing it. In that case, try putting your feet on an ottoman or the couch so that you have something to feel with your heels as you do the acting-as-if pulling down motion of your heels to allow the hamstrings to do more of the work so the quadriceps muscles can quiet down a bit.

Remember that you can watch a video of this activity and all of the activities I'll be teaching you here on my book bonus page: www.theunbreakablebody.com/book-bonus/

Pillar #2: Strong Posture

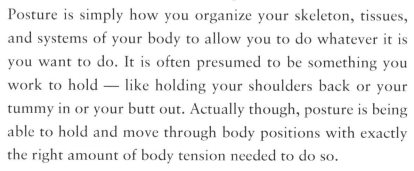

Next, it's time to discuss the Strong Posture Pillar. Folks often think of posture as 'good' or 'bad', as in "I have bad posture." But in reality there's no such thing as good or bad posture. Posture is simply how you organize your skeleton, tissues, and systems of your body to allow you to do whatever it is you want to do. It is often presumed to be something you work to hold — like holding your shoulders back or your tummy in or your butt out. Actually though, posture is being able to hold and move through body positions with exactly the right amount of body tension needed to do so.

That is, you can move fluidly into and through any position you like, and your body organizes itself to do so with ease whether the position you're in is stationary, such as when seated, or when the position is actually a series of positions that make up the movement you are doing, such as when walking or dancing or cleaning up the kitchen after dinner. And, posture is automatic. That is to say, you aren't consciously holding your posture. Sure, you can "pull your shoulders back", but that's not posture. That's just using intentional muscle tension to hold a position. If you let go of the tension in the muscles between your shoulder blades, your shoulders would fall out of that pulled back position you put them in. Posture is simply the state of repose (or 'position') you maintain without extra effort.

One of my favorite mental images to understand a state of repose comes from the world of mechanics, and in particular, stacking and placing objects on angled surfaces. The angle of repose is the steepest angle at which rocks or other objects do not roll down the slope but rather stay put on their own, without any extra support to keep them there.

Your posture is for helping you hold your three chambers of your skeleton, and the rest of your body, in a state of repose without needing extra support to do so. Pulling your shoulders back is akin to putting the rock on a steeper slope so that you then have to put a support under the downhill side of the rock to keep it from tumbling downward. You can't hold that position without intentionally contracting the muscles between your shoulder blades. Not to mention, your skeleton is not held in place *only* by those muscles and so trying to improve posture just by squeezing them, or any other group of muscles, is far too reductionist and isolationist to be useful. In addition, holding your shoulders back, lifting your chin up, or doing any of the other common things you might do to pull yourself into 'good posture' are all forms of rigidness and non-action. They are fixed poses rather than dynamic ones.

Building strong posture is about finding ease in your body, not rigidity. And the path to finding more ease runs through a concept that is now familiar to you — oscillation. Specifically, the ability to rotate the body (which is oscillation in one direction and then back the other direction), to shift from the left side to the right side of the body and back again, and to have access to the full spectrum of muscular tensions available to you.

These oscillations are important for walking, running, going up and down stairs, and doing all of the twisting, reaching, and bending that comes with daily activities, let alone sports. And in a real catch-22, as oscillation is lost, posture becomes more rigid and as posture becomes more rigid, oscillation gets lost.

Dr. Seth Oberst, DPT, sees this in his clinic and he noted it in an article he wrote for my website: "Just watch most anyone walk and you'll notice a lack of symmetrical rotation in the body as people tend to stay stuck on one side (almost always the right)." To restore the ability to rotate, shift, use varying degrees of tension, and have ease in your body, you'll want to restore your ability to oscillate. And the path to being able to oscillate runs through something called neutrality.

The word 'neutrality' may not be familiar, so I want to give you an example to clarify the meaning. Try this with me now... make a fist with your hand. Squeeze the fist as tight and firmly as you can. Really squeeze it! Once it's as squeezed as it can possibly be, can you increase the squeeze-y tension by 25%? Try! Of course, it's a trick — if you're already at max tension, you can't add more tension because there's no more available to you. You're at the endpoint of your tension spectrum when you're at max tension. And when at that endpoint there's no way to go further into tension should you need it.

Now, squeeze your fist a medium amount. Then squeeze a little harder, then a little harder still. Now let go of the squeeze-y tension a bit, then go back up in tension once again. This is the concept of neutrality, where you operate from a state where you can always oscillate toward one end of the spectrum and back towards the other. As Dr. Oberst puts it, "From this state, we can quickly and easily move into all three planes of movement [which means you can rotate, reach, twist and bend as needed] — with the capacity for max tension and max output when necessary."

To build strong posture, you want to create ease in your body, and to create ease you need access to neutrality. We've already talked about something you can do to assist your body in how it is managing tension, that is, whether it's stuck at one end of the spectrum or can move to any point along the entire tension spectrum: breathing. Efficient respiration helps your nervous system to oscillate between the sympathetic and parasympathetic branches, and along with that oscillation comes better management of muscular tension. When you pair efficient respiratory strategies with movement that encourages you to rotate, shift, and find ways to do so with ease, you build strong posture.

I understand that you might be thinking that surely there must be back strengthening exercises you could do to make your posture strong. And while your back muscles may indeed benefit from gaining more strength than they currently have, you know now that posture isn't about any one group of muscles. Remember, your body is always responding to the signals it receives, and the signals are often an interconnected web of many signals rather than just one impacting you. Movement is one way to send a lot of new signals that your body can respond to by organizing your tissues, structures, and systems, in such a way as to grant you stronger posture.

There are many movements you can do to send these signals and I've chosen one that incorporates oscillation, breathing, and an awareness of your entire body, as you do the movement to help you start building strong posture right now. A demonstration of this activity and others are found on the book bonus web page: www.theunbreakablebody.com/book-bonus/

- Sit with your feet flat on the ground and knees bent, keeping your legs hip width apart or slightly closer. An ottoman or low stool works well but if you only have a chair, or you are bed-bound, that works just fine, too. Feel for your sitz bones, which are the bony parts of your butt that are underneath you when you're sitting. Notice your low back: is it arching or pulling you upward? If so, see if you can let that relax, even if that means making it feel more rounded.

- Raise your arms in front of you, parallel with the ground. If your arms can't go that high at the moment, just go as high as you can towards the point where they would be parallel to the ground. With your arms in front of you, shift your hands slightly towards each other so they're a little bit closer together than your shoulders are.

- Take a quiet inhale through your nose and as you exhale gently through your mouth, reach one arm forward so that it moves further forward than the other arm. Notice how if you reach with your right arm, your ribcage turns to the left a little bit. You might also notice that the muscles around the front of your torso contract as you exhale and reach. Keep reaching for as long as you're exhaling. Can you exhale for ten seconds? If not, that's OK, just exhale for however long you can and take note of if the exhale increases over time.

- Once you've completed your exhale, pause for a few seconds and then inhale and bring that arm back to where it started. On your next exhale reach the other arm forward, reaching it for the entire duration of your exhale. Once you've completed that exhale, pause for a few seconds and then inhale and bring that arm back to where it started.

- Continue this alternating arm reaching for a few more reps, and as you do so, start to notice how you're reaching. Is your shoulder rising up into your ear? See if you can let go of whatever is causing the shoulder to rise up. Is your neck or jaw tensing up as you reach? See if you can quiet them down so they are at ease as you reach.

  Do you notice a slight rotating sensation in your ribcage when you reach? If not, see if you can tune into that a bit more by becoming aware of how reaching with one arm causes subtle muscle contractions on the opposite side of your ribcage. Bring your awareness to other areas of your body, your eyes, back, hips, legs, and so on. Can you tell if the tension in any of these areas is increasing? If it is, can you try letting that tension go while you keep up with the reaching motion?

- After you've done several reps of reaching with each arm, bring your arms to rest and take note of how you feel in your body as compared to before you started.

Pillar #3: Strong Feet

Moving on, let's explore the Strong Feet Pillar. When looking at this Pillar, we're looking at the entire foot, ankle and lower leg. Some of the tissues in this area are entirely within the foot itself, while others run from further up your leg, even as far up as the knee.

Your feet influence so much about how you move, by sending your brain copious amounts of information about how you are sensing the ground, how you are organizing movement and balance of your body, , and what the environment you are in is like. All of these signals are being responded to, and even signals that are as seemingly inconsequential as whether you have your weight in your heels or the front of your feet will tell your brain and nervous system something completely different, which can create responses in areas that seem quite distant and separate from your feet.

In speaking with Dr. James Anderson about this, he gave the example of a hot air balloon:

"Imagine a hot air balloon filling up with air, so much so that it lifts off the ground. That's the epitome of having your weight in your toes, you could call it being 'ungrounded'. People who aren't weighting into their heels are lifting up like that balloon. We have muscles that lift us and muscles that ground us — and the people who are un-grounded will be lifting their chest, arching their back, and pushing through the balls of their feet. So, you'd expect to see their calves are tight, their quads and hip flexors are tight, their back is tight, their neck is tight."

This is why it's so important to think of your body as an ecosystem, even when you're tending to one particular Pillar. The Six Pillars are each important and impactful in their own right, and they are important for how they influence other areas of your body. Building strong feet is as much about making your foot muscles stronger and your foot and ankle joints more functional as it is about building your feet, ankles, and lower legs to positively impact the rest of your body.

The first thing to tend to when building strong feet is to expand your awareness of your feet, lower legs, and how you're positioning your body over your feet and lower legs. Most folks don't notice that their toes are pressing heavily into the ground as they stand. Nor do they notice how often they stand with one or both of their knees fully extended and 'locked' in a straight position.

Next time you're standing, notice where your body-weight is in your feet. Then unlock your knees and play with softening them a bit. Then, if you didn't automatically do so when you unlocked your knees, rock your weight backward — not so far that you lose balance and your toes come off the ground, but enough so that you sense your weight in the back of the foot and heel. Bringing awareness to body position is helpful, and you'll also want to tend to how your feet manage the ground as you move through life.

Much of your time on your feet will be spent walking, and perhaps also running. There are quite a few motions and positions your foot will go through with each step you take, including your heel tipping outward and inward, and your foot going from an arched position to a flat position and back to an arched position. Dr. Anderson notes that if you don't have good management of your heel, or you have high arches or flat feet, finding the ability to optimally navigate through the foot positions needed for walking and running gait can be difficult, which can create accommodations further 'upstream' in your body, as the nervous system adjusts tension and positions elsewhere to deal with what's lacking down below. And so, the next thing to do to help your feet is to help them access each position and motion needed for gait. In the ancient past, your ancestors walked barefoot on natural surfaces. They traveled through tall, soft grass and over soft dirt and sand. These natural environments were wonderful for meeting your ancestors' feet with their natural contours. Just picture how when you walk barefoot on the beach, your foot sinks in and is met by the sand at all of the curves and contours of your foot.

Your body responds favorably when its contours are met and supported, so it's a real bummer that we all live in modern society now with its hard floors and concrete ground. Just kidding — it's nice to live in modern times — but you're going to need to help your nervous system and body appreciate modern life by assisting your foot in feeling met and supported where those contours are.

When your foot meets hard ground unsupported, as in when walking barefoot or in flimsy shoes on hard unnatural surfaces, your brain and body will have to accommodate for the fact that the support is not there. This can contribute to responses like increased muscle tension and changes to your gait pattern, which can mean that tissues that aren't built for the job you're asking them to do now have to do that job excessively.

Appropriate footwear for the environment your foot is in is how you provide the contour support your foot needs so that better information can get to your nervous system and better responses can then come from it. If you are walking on a soft, natural, surface like sand or tall grass, your foot will be met and there's no need for a middle man to meet the foot's contours. A shoe that has minimal support, often advertised as a minimalist shoe, will be just fine. If, however, you're walking on a hard surface like concrete, wood or tiled floors, or anything similarly unnatural, take note of the lack of contour support in those types of floors and use a shoe that can create the contour support that your foot wants but isn't getting from the floor. As Dr. Anderson puts it, "bring the beach to your foot."

When you're looking for footwear that meets your foot's contours and can help your foot handle the motions and positions that are required for optimal gait, there are a few common traits to look for:

1. They have a sturdy heel, and not the heel like the one on a high-heeled shoe. A sturdy heel is one that wraps around the back of your heel and serves as a firm support for the back of your foot. To know if it's a sturdy heel, try pushing down on it. If it collapses, it's not sturdy.

2. The footwear supports your midfoot, where the arch of your foot is. To know if the shoe has a supportive midfoot, try bending the shoe in half. If it bends in the middle, it's not a supportive midfoot. The bend you seek in the shoe is going to be closer towards the front of the shoe.

3. You want the shoe to stay attached to your foot with laces or a buckle. When your shoe isn't attached to your foot, as with a slip-on or flip-flop sandal, your foot muscles have to change how they operate as you go through that gait cycle and can once again create accommodations you might not prefer long-term.

4. You want room for your toes to spread out as you step. Look at the shoe from a top-down perspective and then look at your foot from the same perspective. If the shoe narrows more than your foot does as you look

from the front of your foot where the ball joints of the toes are out toward the tips of your toes, it's not likely to give your toes enough room to spread as you walk.

All this talk of footwear might make you think that building your Strong Feet Pillar is just about applying external signals to your body, but that couldn't be further from the truth. Internal signals like resistance training exercises and mobility drills are of the utmost importance when building your Strong Feet Pillar.

Your feet and lower legs have muscles, joints and other soft tissues, all of which respond to forces being placed on them, just like the rest of your body does. And those muscles and joints have jobs they are built for, but when those tissues and joints don't have the capacity to work as they are built to, your body will accommodate you and find another way. This leads to other tissues and joints being called upon to do more work or to do jobs they're not as well suited for.

And yet, resistance training exercises and mobility expanding drills often stop at the knee. This doesn't make any sense. Use internal signals to teach your foot and lower leg tissues to respond such that they become stronger and more capable of generating and receiving force without failure.

Here is an activity you can do to start building your Strong Feet Pillar. A demonstration of this activity and others are found on the book bonus web page: www.theunbreakablebody.com/book-bonus/

This can be done sitting or standing (sitting is easier than standing when starting out). It's also preferably done without shoes or socks on in the beginning, as there is a measurable impact from being able to see what you're doing.

- With your feet flat on the ground and facing forward, press your little toes into the ground while you lift only your big toes up. Keep all of the small toes on the ground. Set the big toes back down.
- Then lift only your little toes while pressing your big toes on the ground. Set the little toes back down. Alternate back and forth between these two lifts.
- If you notice that it's dang near impossible for you to do this initially, you're not alone. Of the people I've taught this to over the years, about 90% have really struggled with it at first. But 100% of those who stuck with it, despite struggling, eventually became able to do the activity.
- Notice if your body is trying to move other parts of your foot and ankle to accommodate the motion you're trying to do with your toes. If your ankles are caving inward or shifting outward, try to quiet that down and allow the motion to stay within the foot. If your shin bone is shifting backward to "help out", you may hold your lower leg to keep it stationary as you practice.
- If you cannot figure out how to get only the big or only the little toes up, use your hand to hold down

the toes you do not want to move while using your other hand to help lift the toe you do want to move. Then, see if you can find the muscles within your foot that hold the toe positions in place and try letting go with your hands. At first, it may feel like there are no muscles that connect to your toes in that position, but over time, you'll develop a stronger sensory connection to the right muscles for the activity.

Pillars #4 and 5: Mobile Hips and Mobile Shoulders

Next, we're on to the two 'Mobility' Pillars — Mobile Hips and Mobile Shoulders. I've combined these two together here because the concepts of building mobility in each are so similar.

Both the hips and the shoulders have a ball and socket joint, which is where the ball-shaped surface of one rounded bone fits into the cup-like depression of another bone. (Your shoulder also has the scapula bone that is made to move along the ribcage.) Having ball and socket joints means those joints are built to have a large degree of motion. In fact, your hips and shoulders are the two most mobile joints in your body. As such, improving the motion of these two joints is a primary objective.

It pays to understand first how joint motion, or mobility,

is increased because you'll apply this to both your hips and your shoulders. And increasing the amount of mobility you have in your hips and shoulders means you'll have more movements you're able to do, which is great, given how necessary your hips and shoulders are for so many of the movements required in life:

- Reaching
- Squatting
- Sitting down
- Standing up
- Walking
- Picking something up
- Carrying something
- Doing workouts and sports

All these movements require that your hips and shoulders be able to move (and having them move *well* sure does make it easier and more enjoyable to do all of these things).

If you've ever felt tightness or restriction in your shoulder or hips, you're not alone. Nearly everyone will, at some point, realize that the amount of mobility they have in their hips or shoulders is less than the amount they need to do the things they love.

Mobility refers to how much passive range of motion and active range of motion you have. Passive range of motion demonstrates how far your tissues will allow you to move, while active range of motion demonstrates how much movement your muscles are strong enough to control.

Passive range of motion is the amount of movement through which your joint can move when you are *not* actively contracting muscles to move the limb through its range of motion. If you're working with a physical therapist and they take your arm and lift it up as high as it will go while you relax, that is passive range of motion. Similarly, if you place your hand on a wall and turn away from it to stretch your chest muscles, that too is passive range of motion. Other examples of passive range of motion include using a stretching strap to pull your limb into a position, using the weight of gravity to stretch you as you fold over at the waist and reach for your toes, and having a partner to pull you further into a stretch.

Active range of motion is the amount of movement through which you can voluntarily move your joint through *without* assistance from another body part, person or device. If instead of the physical therapist lifting your arm up, you raise your arm up by using the muscles of that arm, that is active range of motion. Other examples include using your muscles to pull your toes and top of your foot up towards your shins, to pull your knee and thigh towards your chest, and to twist your torso around as you'd do when sitting in a chair and needing to reach for something behind you, such as in the backseat of a car. Anytime you contract your muscles to flex, straighten, or rotate your joint, that is you using your active range of motion.

When you use your passive or active range of motion, you'll eventually come to an endpoint. An endpoint is the point at which you can't go any further with your range of motion. It often feels like a stopping point where your body is telling you "that's it, that's the end." But often, you're not actually at your physiological endpoint, but rather, more of a functional end point where there is more range of motion *available* to you but not yet *accessible* to you.

A common reason for this limitation is the joint capsule itself not having enough 'work space' in it. A joint needs room to move in its home, the joint capsule. To picture what it's like to not have enough room to move, imagine putting on a jacket that is much too small for you and zipping it up. Your arms are stuck at an outward angle because the jacket is so tight you can't bring them to your sides. The body of the jacket is holding your torso such that you can't really round your back if you were to try to bend over and look down at something. Trying to go through your day like this, doing all of the activities you normally do, would be a real challenge.

Similarly, when your joint has lost work space, it can't move in all the ways it's built to move. Lost work space most commonly develops when an injury doesn't heal correctly or fully, or when you stop using that joint through its full and complete range of motion on a regular basis. Remember learning that your body prioritizes what it should maintain and provide upkeep for based on how consistently you're using it?

Take your shoulder as an example. The glenohumeral joint of your shoulder is the ball and socket joint where the arm meets the body, and it's built to move your arm through a significant range of motion. Daily life commonly includes movements like reaching into cabinets, brushing your hair, and getting dressed. While those can be quite painful if you're experiencing an injury that limits your shoulder range of motion, they're still not even the full scope of range of motion a glenohumeral joint is built to move through. And so, if you don't use your full range of motion regularly, your body de-prioritizes the upkeep of that range of motion.

This issue of disuse is not just limited to the joint and its joint capsule either. When you don't move your limbs so that your joints go through their full and complete range of motion consistently, the muscles that lie in the area of that joint also are affected. As you know now, movement teaches your body's muscles how to generate and receive forces which in turn makes those tissues stronger and better. Movement also teaches your nervous system that you have control over the various lengths and tensions your muscle goes through as you move. If your nervous system hasn't learned to allow you to lengthen or shorten a muscle to a certain point so as to flex or rotate your joint fully, it can perceive that as being an unsafe range of motion to enter. This might feel like you simply don't have more range of motion beyond your current endpoint. But, that's often not the case.

There are two ways in which you can teach your nervous

system that it is safe to enter a range of motion — first, demonstrate to your nervous system that you are regularly entering as much of your range of motion as possible. Or more succinctly, use it or lose it. If you regularly use as much range of motion as you currently have, you'll fend off the loss of range of motion that comes with disuse and you'll capture a range of motion that is at the edges of where your current access lies.

Second, teach your nervous system that it's safe to enter greater and greater ranges of motion by becoming stronger. And in particular, become stronger at the current endpoint of your range of motion. As you move your joint through its range of motion to its endpoint, some of the muscles that are helping to move that joint are becoming more lengthened while the opposing muscles are becoming more shortened.

Here's a quick example to illustrate this: in order to lift your leg up and over something, whether it's the edge of the bathtub or a high step you're using in a workout to step up onto, you need to flex at your hip crease to lift your leg up. (You will likely also externally rotate your hip as you do this, but we'll just focus on hip flexion at this time.) As you lift your leg up towards you so that your hip and knee come towards your torso, the flexor muscles on the front of your hip get shorter while the glutes on the back of your hip get longer. At some point, your hip will run into its endpoint and you'll feel like you're at the end of your range of motion. If that is before you get to the height necessary to step over or onto whatever is in front of you, you'll have to either accommodate yourself by using other muscles and joints to help you, or you'll just have to not step over or onto the object.

But the muscles on the front and back of your hip often have the potential to lengthen or shorten further, thus allowing you to flex your hip further and pull your leg up higher with ease — they are just unable to generate enough force to do so. In order to get them strong enough to do so, you need to contract the muscles in those positions and at those lengths. That is, learn to contract the muscles of the front and back of your hip when they are in that position that shortens one side and lengthens the other where you currently aren't strong enough to go further.

Dr. Andreo Spina, founder of Functional Range Systems, shares this on the subject in his lecture on increasing range of motion for students taking his Functional Range Conditioning seminar:

> "Show your nervous system that you can contract the tissue in question in a specific position at a specific joint angle. In turn, your nervous system will then grant you a small increase in the degrees of range of motion you can access."

That small increase grants you more length, which grants you more range of motion, and as Dr. Spina goes on to say, "as you progress into greater and greater degrees of range of motion, we are systematically teaching our nervous system to be strong at these small, consistent intervals." Thus, your nervous system learns how to control a new range of motion, you get more range of motion, and you get stronger in that range of motion. This then allows you to move more freely and with greater control.

Finally, there can be other reasons why tissues and joints can be tight-feeling, including physiological limitations, such as the joint being structured in a way that you can't move any further with that joint without running into bone, neuro-muscular diseases like MS that come with symptoms like muscle tightness, and even your average cold or flu can make your muscles and joints feel more stiff. Remember that your body is an ecosystem — full of systems and parts and things your nervous system is responding to, and one solution doesn't solve all issues.

And so, the very common misunderstanding that if something feels 'tight' it needs to be stretched, isn't accurate at all. Your body is always responding to the signals it receives, and so a tight muscle is a body response to information your nervous system is processing and using to decide how much 'tone' or tension that muscle should hold. Whether it's your joint itself that feels stiff and tight, or it feels like you've got a tight muscle somewhere, the tension is there for a reason. While a gentle stretch might feel great (and it's by no means bad to do) you might just find a greater sense of ease in your muscle and joint with something that does not resemble a stretch at all!

Before we do the exercises for Mobile Hips and Mobile Shoulders, we need to acknowledge foam rollers, massage tools, and other similar self-massage items that are commonly included in the list of 'things that improve mobility'…

The benefit of these is that they are a form of self-care that most people will gladly spend the time to do because they don't require much effort and they make you feel good. That is not to be discounted in the slightest because, quite frankly, anything that helps a person feel more relaxed in modern life is a good thing.

However, self-massage tools do not change your mobility, nor do they "break up knots and adhesions" or eliminate scar tissue. The force and duration required to do those things is far beyond what you can do with a foam roller or massage gun. So if you're going to use self-massage tools, just know that they aren't impacting your long-term tissue quality or your joint mobility. But if they feel nice and you want to spend the time using them, then have at it.

Here is an activity you can do — not stretching! — to start building the active range of motion in your hips and shoulders. A demonstration of this activity and others are found on the book bonus web page: www.theunbreakablebody.com/book-bonus/

First, the shoulder activity:

- Lay on your side with a pillow for support under your head. Your bottom arm can be resting any way that is comfortable for you. Set your body so that your knees are pulled up to a right angle with your hips, and your spine is in a straight line (as opposed to how you might curl up into a ball when sleeping). Try not to move any part of your body other than the limb we're doing the activity with. Common parts that might want to move are your head and neck muscles, and your spine and torso.

- Rest your top arm on the ground in front of you so that your palm is flat resting on the ground and your elbow is straight. We're going to be drawing a circle with your arm: imagine a round wall clock and picture that your arm is pointing towards the nine on the clock. Begin by moving your arm towards the twelve on the clock; this will be near your head. Keep your elbow totally straight, and bring your arm as close to that twelve position as you can. You might get stopped before you hit that position due to tightness or restriction, and that's OK, just make note of it as something to work on. Or, you might get your bicep to touch your head because you got the arm all the way to the twelve position.

- From there, turn your wrist so that your pinkie finger points to the sky, and then continue the turning-up motion so that your palm starts to turn towards the sky as well.

- Once you've turned your arm and hand, start moving your arm towards the three position on the clock.

Remember to keep your elbow straight as you keep reaching behind you. As you move your arm toward the three position, keep rotating your palm and arm and see if you can get your palm to face the ceiling again when you get to the three position. It's OK if you can't get that much twist yet, just get as far as you can.

- As you pass the three position on the clock, continue on so that your arm comes towards the six position on the clock and then around to your legs and to the starting point where it began, holding onto that twisting motion with your arm. You've just explored your current active range of motion for your glenohumeral joint of your shoulder. Switch sides and repeat the movement with the other arm.

Now onto the hip activity:

- To do the hip activity, start on your hands and knees on the ground or on a bed. If it hurts to be on your wrists, you can make fists instead of having flat palms. Try not to move any part of your body other than the limb we're doing the activity with. Again, common parts that might want to move are your head and neck muscles and your spine, torso, and pelvis.
- Begin by lifting your heel toward your glute on whichever leg you're doing first. By pulling your heel toward your glute you have just flexed your knee. Now, keep your knee flexed like that and pull that leg forward so

that your knee comes towards your chest.

- Once you've drawn your knee as close to your chest as you can without moving any other part of your body, lift your leg out to the side of your body, as high as you can without bending your arms or moving any other part of your body. Try to have your knee and your foot parallel or close to it as you're holding it out to the side of your body.

- Next, start to lift your foot higher than your knee (you might need to drop your knee down a bit to achieve this) and begin pulling your leg around towards your backside, as if you were drawing the edge of a circle with your knee as you go from the knee being at your side to now being behind you.

- Once you've brought your leg all the way around so that it's now directly behind you, lower it down to rest next to the non-moving leg. Then reverse the motion to go back the way you came, first by lifting the leg up directly behind you so that your knee is flexed and your heel is close to your glutes.

- From there, turn your thigh so your knee points outward. Start to pull your thigh out and around, again as if you are drawing the edge of a circle, to bring your thigh to the position it was in previously, held out to the side of your body.

- Once your thigh is out at your side, pull it underneath you so your knee is as close to your chest as you can get without moving any other part of your body. Then relax. You've just explored your current active range of motion for your hip joint. Switch sides and repeat the movement with the other leg.

Pillar #6: Strong Glutes

Finally, we find our way to the Strong Glutes Pillar. Your glutes are helping you every day, far more than just to keep the backside of your pants up. They have several important jobs to do to aid you in movement, including extending your hip, shifting your leg outward away from your midline, and externally and internally rotating the hip joint. You'll need these motions should you want to walk, run, get up from a chair or crouched position, get out of your car, go up and down stairs, and do much of what you need to do in daily life activities, not to mention when you take up exercise, sports, or other extracurricular activities.

The Strong Glutes Pillar begins first with ensuring you can find and contract your glute muscles. You might think that if we are trying to 'find' your glute muscles that perhaps you've 'lost' them, or that they have 'forgotten' how to contract. Neither of these are true. This type of language comes from a time when a popular (but inaccurate) way to describe sub-optimal glute function was 'glute amnesia'. It is impossible for your glutes to forget how to contract, but it *is* possible for your glute muscles to become weak.

And muscle weakness does not develop merely because you don't do enough resistance training to build muscular strength. I'm speaking first of simply a lack of usage of the glute muscles for their intended purpose. As I mentioned, your glute muscles are meant to contract as you do all sorts of daily life activities, like walking and using the stairs. However, in order for your glute muscles to engage fully and effectively in those daily activities, there's something you need to do which is often lost somewhere along the way: oscillation.

Yes, once again, oscillation shows up in the body story. We've talked about it with the two branches of the autonomic nervous system, and with your ability to find strong posture, and now we're talking about it with regard to building strong glutes. There is meant to be a natural oscillation of your bodyweight as you move through your gait — whether walking or running — where you shift and rotate your bodyweight from the left side of your body to right side and back again. This transfer of bodyweight aids in propelling you forward. Even when not in motion, you're meant to have the ability to oscillate your bodyweight between your left side and your right, standing more on one side, then standing more on the other, and your glute muscles aid you in doing this.

However, due to a number of factors including how you breathe, past injuries, and the fact that the human body is simply not symmetrical, it is common to develop a body accommodation where you shift more to one side than the other. Recall that Dr. Seth Oberst quote from when we talked about posture, here it is again: "Just watch most anyone walk and you'll notice a lack of symmetrical rotation in the body as people tend to stay stuck on one side (almost always the right)." This stuck-ness to one side is due in part to the glutes not participating as fully as possible. Your glutes contribute heavily to getting you propelled from one foot to the other and in doing so, they shift your body weight from one side to the other. *Or they should.*

Another common body accommodation for weak glutes is to use more of your hip flexor muscles on the front of your hip crease and your low back muscles to assist in doing the job that the glutes are built to do. And, the more you practice these accommodations, the more ingrained and unconscious they become and the more likely you are to depend on that particular accommodation over time.

Remember that accommodations are not bad, but they do come with consequences, and those consequences become a problem when they detract from you being able to do the things you want to do and feeling how you want to feel. One of the consequences of not oscillating your bodyweight from one side to the other as effectively or efficiently as you should is that the glute muscles become weak because they're not being engaged as fully as possible. This impacts not only your glute muscles, but can also impact the rest of your skeleton and how you stack it because nothing in your body ecosystem works in isolation.

For example, weakness in your glute muscles might show up as irritation in your hip muscles or an achy feeling in your low back as they do more work to take care of what the glutes are not doing. And so, a natural starting place for building strong glutes is to ensure that they are working in the manner they're meant to in basic, everyday activities.

You can also use glute strength as a proxy for other aspects of your health and wellbeing. Your glutes are made up of a complex of muscles that make them the biggest and strongest in your body. If the glutes are weak, there's a good chance you also have muscle weakness elsewhere in your body, which means there is a good chance you have less overall muscle mass.

Muscle mass is incredibly influential to your health. Your ability to manage your blood glucose levels, your overall metabolic rate, your bone density, your risk of falling, and your ability to recover after surgery, are all influenced by the amount of muscle mass you carry. In addition, "weakness of the gluteus maximus has been implicated in numerous injury types such as anterior knee pain, anterior cruciate ligament injuries… hamstring strains, and ankle sprains."[26]

An injury isn't just a problem in the obvious sense — it

26 Buckthorpe, M., Stride, M., & Della Villa, F., (2019 July 14). Assessing And Treating Gluteus Maximus Weakness - A Clinical Commentary. *International Journal of Sports Physical Therapy* 14(4): 655–669

also has the potential to be a much larger problem for your overall quality of life and health. When you sustain an injury, it can completely alter how much you move in a given day, and moving less can start a snowball effect leading to a loss of muscle mass and fitness, a loss of cardiovascular health, a loss of balance and proprioception, and a decline in cognition and mood. Avoiding injury when possible is ideal, and if your glutes are strong, there are more movements you can do, positions you can get into, and forces you can handle.

In addition, building strong glutes is not just about making sure your glutes work well for you as you do your daily activities and for your overall health, although both those things seem like pretty great reasons to build strong glutes. You're also going to need strong glutes for the sports and adventures you want to partake in (naturally, this is also true for the rest of your muscles in your body). It's been shown that "strength training can lead to enhanced long-term and short-term endurance capacity both in well-trained individuals and highly trained top-level endurance athletes."[27]

A well-designed strength training program includes ample amounts of work for the glute muscles, and these benefits are seen again and again as you look at various sports and the benefits gained when an individual takes up a resistance training program.

---

27   Aagaard, P., & Andersen, J. L. (2010). Effects of strength training on endurance capacity in top-level endurance athletes. *Scandinavian journal of medicine & science in sports*. 20 Suppl 2, 39-47. https://doi.org/10.1111/j.1600-0838.2010.01197.x

Here is an activity you can do to start building your strong glutes. If you'd like to use a chair for support, by all means do so. A demonstration of this activity and others are found on the book bonus web page: www.theunbreakablebody.com/book-bonus/

- Take a pillow and stand next to a wall that does not have anything hanging on it. Stand with the wall at your side so that your shoulder is next to the wall. If you're using a chair for support, place it in front of you so that you can put your hands on the back of it. Place the pillow against the hip that is next to the wall and close the distance between you and the wall so that the pillow can be held in place by your hip and the wall. You might need to fold it in half if it's not thick enough.

- Look down at your feet and ensure both are pointing straight forward. Relax your knees so that they are unlocked but not bent. Notice your body positioning and find the best stack of your head, torso, hips, legs, and feet, *without* doing any of the following to achieve it: arching your back, puffing your chest out, or sticking your butt out to find the stack.

- Bring your awareness to the foot that is further from the wall and feel for the arch of your foot and your big toe ball joint. See if you can increase your awareness of those areas pressing into the floor. Let the foot closest to the wall be light as you're going to be lifting it off the ground shortly.

- Begin to press more firmly into the pillow that is between you and the wall, by shifting your weight towards the wall. Rather than just leaning into the wall casually, do this shifting with intent by increasing the pressure of your foot pressing down into the ground to assist you shifting into the wall. Notice how your glute muscles on that outer leg start contracting more firmly as you press more into the wall and into the ground.

- Raise the foot closest to the wall slightly off the ground and continue pressing firmly into the pillow. Can you smoosh the pillow firmly into the wall without needing to flex your low back, your neck, or any other part of you other than the grounded leg that is driving you into the wall? Feel your glute muscles working to hold you there. Hold for ten to twenty seconds. Then relax and turn around to face the other way and repeat with the other leg.

Building Your Six Pillars

These Six Pillars — Strong Torso, Strong Posture, Strong Feet, Mobile Hips and Shoulders, and Strong Glutes — are the base of support for your Unbreakable body. As you know by now, becoming Unbreakable is not about following some exact plan that works for everyone. One size does not fit all in this world, and nowhere is that more true than in your care of your body, mind, and spirit.

Even in my Unbreakable Body training program, you get to take the program and tailor it to suit you, rather than forcing yourself to fit it. And, as you also know, building and maintaining your Six Pillars is a lifelong thing, so once you've identified exercises and activities that build your Pillars, you can inject them into anything you're doing for your body.

For instance, many of my students will take my program that builds all six of the Pillars, and then when they decide to go onto something else, they'll keep their favorite and most impactful Pillar exercises as extras to include in their next workout program. You can also overlay the Six Pillars on top of things you're already doing, perhaps a weekly yoga class, triathlons, or a fitness class you're taking at the gym, and use it to double-check that you're getting what you need to keep your base strong.

To figure out how much you need to tend to each of your Six Pillars, first think of your body and any aches or pains you're dealing with. Those are usually great indicators for you to know that attention is needed, perhaps in the area where the ache is felt, or in another area of your body that is accommodating you in some way.

Then think about basic movements you need your body to do every day that are required for you to function on your own, such as putting on pants, sitting on the toilet, reaching for stuff on the shelves, walking to the car, and so on. Do you have enough capacity in each of the Pillars to accomplish these things? Then think about anything that you'd like to be able to do that's beyond your daily basics, like extracurricular activities, sports, or adventures you want to go on. This list could include things like wanting to be able to throw your dog's ball countless times in the park after work without having your shoulder give out long before the pup is tired. It could also be the adult ice hockey league you like to play in where you want to feel solid and strong. Or it could be that big goal you have to do a cross-country bike ride which is going to require a lot of training and you want your body to hold up to it. And finally, think back to your vision of what becoming Unbreakable looks and feels like to you. What do your Six Pillars need to help you embody what you envision?

These four categories — where your body is currently speaking to you through aches and pains, basic movement capacity requirements for life, the 'extracurriculars' you want to participate in, and your Unbreakable vision — are a good metric to use to determine if your body has enough of what it needs to do these things you need and want to do. In addition, I've included a mini-self assessment of the Six Pillars on the book bonus page.

No matter where you're starting from, one thing is for sure: the Six Pillars always meet you where you are and support you as you move forward from there on your journey to becoming Unbreakable. And as you build your Six Pillars, you create a groundswell of capacity and confidence that makes you sit up and take notice of yourself. When you can say, "Wow, I *can* actually change how my body feels and moves," it inevitably leads to, "I wonder what else I could make an impact on?"

If you're new to exercise, it's worth working with a coach or following a program designed by a coach. Doing the program will help you get on the right track with results, and it will also help you learn a few things about program design simply by watching how the program is laid out for you. You can then take this knowledge and put it to use if you want to design your own program in the future. My Unbreakable Body workout program is a perfect next-step to implement what you've learned in the book and to learn how to create and tailor your own training program in the future.

Next, remember that forces on your body are how your body's tissues change. And the more specific the force (signal) on your tissues, the more specific the adaptation (response). When you're trying to build a stronger body and greater mobility, you'll want to focus on doing some form of resistance training. Resistance training can be done with added resistance, such as with barbells, dumbbells, resistance bands, and even household objects. But it can also be done with just your bodyweight, too, so if you don't have fitness equipment, don't let that stop you from getting started. The objective is to place an amount of force on your tissues that is appropriate for your current tissue tolerance, and helps to move you in the direction you're trying to go.

Remember when we talked about the zones of tissue tolerance? For beginners, simply doing a lot of work in your zone of homeostasis is a great starting point because it builds your tolerance to exercise and helps to form the habit of exercising regularly. This means doing a lot of movements in your exercise program that are currently achievable. Too often, folks make it too hard too quickly, often because there is a misperception that for exercise to 'work', it should feel hard.

There is a principle in exercise known as the SAID Principle, which is an acronym that stands for Specific Adaptations to Imposed Demands. While it's true that dipping your toes across the envelope of function into that realm of supraphysiologic overload is a useful tool to build your capacity, if the forces you ask your body to respond to are so great that they are well beyond what you can currently do, you're not going to get the adaptations you desire. You want to impose demands on your tissues that your tissues can respond to favorably. Eventually, you can start using what is called the Overload Principle, where you gradually make the exercises harder so that your body will continue to adapt.

But if you are just starting out, start with something more simple and easy to do, then work up to making it more complex and difficult. Start with a shorter session, then increase the amount of work you're doing so the session time increases. Start with exercising at a frequency that you can easily manage, then increase the amount you do over time. There's an abundance of research that has looked into whether or not there is an ideal way (how many days a week, how long of a session, etc.) to do a resistance training program, and what often shakes out in the end is that two or three times a week is effective for most goals, and what actually matters more is that you're presenting your tissues enough of a demand that they can respond and continue to adapt.

But what if you don't have two or three days a week to devote to resistance training? Being an Unbreakable human is about always finding a way to continue the forward progress of your journey, which is why it's so important that you know about the Signal/Response Principle, and to build your ability to use curious compassion as you explore and experiment. Your body might not respond with as many strength gains if you do resistance training once a week, but the question I always ask is: isn't that still better than just bagging the whole thing until you've got time to do it two to three times a week?

Momentum is built on consistency and momentum in one area of your life tends to extend into other areas of your life. Even small weekly wins in the consistency department help to anchor other habits you engage in to support your Unbreakable body.

Speaking of other habits, building your Six Pillars is not just relegated to your physical training time. Recall that we discussed in the last chapter how your daily life includes an abundance of opportunities to send signals to your body that impart forces in the tissues that your tissues will respond to, both in including little 'movement breaks' in your day, and even in the miniscule moments that are so routine you do them without thinking.

Here's an example of how I bring the Strong Feet Pillar into my day. Every person who comes to my house comments that I have a rock on my kitchen floor. "Well, wouldn't you like to have a foot massage while you make coffee in the morning?" I reply. The rock is there because I can't miss it when I go to make coffee. It's out and ready for doing a bit of self massage on my feet as the coffee brews, and I can do it mindlessly. It serves as the tiniest reminder to think of my feet as I go through the day, which might manifest as doing foot strengthening exercises later, or doing a short little calf stretch as I wait in the grocery checkout line.

Here are a few more examples of creative ways to make your daily life more supportive of your Unbreakable body:

- If you notice that when work gets stressful, you start breathing more shallowly, set a reminder on your phone that says "breathe completely" and take a minute to do just that.
- If you catch yourself carrying your bag on one shoulder all the time, switch it to the other one.
- If you're waiting for your leftovers to heat up for

dinner, do a few reps of a movement that you learned to help your shoulders explore their range of motion (both the book bonus and my full Unbreakable Body program have options).

- If you always sit in a chair, spend some time sitting on the floor. And if you can't sit on the floor, try simply sitting on your bed as if you are sitting on the floor — and then make a note to explore and experiment with exercises and activities that could help you become able to sit on the floor.

- Instead of scrolling on your phone in the evening, spend five minutes of that time moving each of your joints through their range of motion. (Again, see my book bonus or Unbreakable Body program for exercise options.)

- Look at the kinds of shoes and clothes you wear and decide if they assist your body in getting what it needs to move optimally.

Your environment is going to differ from someone else's and the point is not to lament what you don't have but rather to make it work with what you do have. That's why I so strongly encourage you to explore, experiment, and curate. Because if you wait for all the 'right' stuff to be in your environment to start building your Unbreakable body, you're going to be waiting a long time. So get going, and make life in your body-ecosystem as hospitable as possible.

CHAPTER 15:

Building Your Unbreakable Life

A t the age of 33, I found myself setting a proverbial match to my entire life and burning to the ground all that I had created thus far, so I could build something new.

The life I burned down appeared nice enough, even to me for a time. I owned a gym that was flourishing and which gave me a suitable salary. I had clients and friends who I thoroughly enjoyed. I had a sense of routine which I'd grown accustomed to. A favorite coffee shop where they knew my order as soon as I walked in the door. A favorite walk to a favorite place to watch the sunset. I had all my favorites and I made sure that they filled my days.

But one night, I was writing in my journal, doing my usual free flow writing to get all the random thoughts out of my head and onto the paper. This has always been one of the best ways for me to see what I actually think, feel, and believe, because the thoughts can get out onto the paper before my thinking brain has a chance to catch them and form an opinion.

On the page I wrote: *I am here to help people become strong in their bodies so they can create a life beyond anything they had ever dreamed was possible. And I can't do that for myself here.*

What the hell. I had never thought that second sentence before. But there it was, and as I read it back, I felt the truth of it in my bones. I snapped to attention. A decade of learning to listen to the responses my body gave me made me certain I needed to take notice. And even though this response was coming from the imprecise place in my body where my soul resides, the resonance of it was impossible to ignore.

I immediately started exploring my ecosystems to identify what signals my soul was so clearly responding to. I combed through my inner ecosystem, including my body and what it got to do each day, as well as my beliefs, fears, needs, and greatest desires. I took stock of my outer ecosystem that I lived in every day, including my work, where I lived, and how I spent my time. I collected data about what was working in my life, and what might not be. I started pondering what wasn't in my life that maybe should be. And then it hit me.

All these people, places, and things in my life were lovely. But I'd become as much of Me as I could be with these people, in this place, doing these things. I could either continue on with what I'd built for my life thus far, sacrificing the Me I'm meant to become in the process. Or, I could get to work making moves to find the signals of a new place and a new way of life — and new experiences — that would allow me to become the Me I didn't even know yet that I could be.

It wasn't long before I hauled out to Utah to visit some friends and explore whether a relocation out there might be the right move for me. On my final night there, we hiked up to a rocky outcrop overlooking the city, called Pete's Rock, to watch the sunset and I thought, "Yup, I'm doin' it." I decided that night to torch the life I knew, close my gym, let go of the lease on my adorable little rental house, and rebuild all of it in a new place and an entirely new way.

I had no idea what would lie ahead but I knew three things for certain:

One, I could trust myself with this big decision because I'd spent years practicing listening to my body's responses and making decisions based on them to build and care for my Unbreakable body.

Two, I could tolerate any and all potential outcomes of my choice, even if they were negative, because in a decade of building my Unbreakable body, I was well versed in making everything work for me. Whether by finding the lesson about what not to do next time, or by learning something about myself and the world around me, I knew that any outcome is more useful than the outcome of never trying.

And three, I must listen to my inner voice and ignore everyone else's opinion about what I should do, because while they might be well-meaning, they do not know better than me what is right for me. I'd built my personal autonomy, and it sure came in handy when my soul decided to speak up.

In Dr. Christopher Ryan's book, *Civilized To Death*, personal autonomy is a theme that comes up frequently as he explores whether or not civilization has been a good thing for humans. At one point, he references the notes of Daniel Everett, a linguist who spent more than two decades living with and studying a remote Amazonian tribe called the Pirahã, and one note stood out in particular to me. Writes Everett:

> "Since my first night among them, I have been impressed with their patience, their happiness, and their kindness. This pervasive happiness is hard to explain though I believe the Pirahã are so confident and secure in their ability to handle anything that their environment throws at them that they can enjoy whatever comes their way."[28]

---

28   Ryan, C (2019). *Civilized To Death: The Price of Progress*. New York City, New York, USA: Avid Reader Press / Simon & Schuster

Dr. Christopher Ryan uses this note as a flag waving in the breeze to indicate that us modern humans don't feel as secure as the Pirahã, because we've created an environment where the things you need to be able to trust yourself to handle are no longer simple issues like predators or a drought — they are complex and mentally worrisome things like tax audits and recessions.

This is true: modern environments create far more opportunities to find yourself in a perpetually stressed state with your sympathetic nervous system ramped up and ready to fight or flee. Our ancestors would have only tapped into that state when there was imminent danger and they'd have exited from the stressful state as soon as the danger had passed. But if this is what existing in the modern world means, wouldn't you like to cultivate more of the confident, ready-for-anything state that the Pirahã exude?

If modern life is going to throw some nasty stuff your way — and let's be honest, even if you never receive an audit notice from the IRS, something equally unnerving will come your way sooner or later — wouldn't you like to know that you have a well of empowered confidence and self-trust to draw from as you handle it? And forget the big scary stuff you may have to handle — wouldn't you like to simply feel more at peace amidst the chaos of the modern world?

You most likely do not live deep in the Amazon like the Pirahã, but you can cultivate your own kind of secure internal state where you can handle anything your environment throws at you.

This is what becoming Unbreakable is all about. It's so much more than building your physical body. I know we've covered a lot about that up to this point — because if your body doesn't feel how you want it to feel and can't do what you want it to do, it's going to influence many other areas of your life.

And when you build your physical body to be Unbreakable, you naturally also build attributes like self-sufficiency, confidence and fortitude, which help you in other areas of life. So while building your Unbreakable body, with an emphasis on the physical body part, is of the utmost importance, these last few pages are dedicated to the aspects of becoming Unbreakable that have nothing to do with your physical body.

As we wrap up this book, I want to share a sentiment expressed by an Unbreakable human named Anu, who crossed my path through my Unbreakable Body workout program. These words express in a lovely way the nature of how the physical body intertwines with your experience of living in the world:

> "An Unbreakable body is shaped by resilient posture and grounded by strong feet, mobile hips and torso that bend with gratitude, open shoulders to welcome opportunities, and wild heart and fiery glutes to move and groove with love and compassion." — Anu

You don't have to burn down your life as you know it to get a life like what Anu is describing. Far from it, in fact. But you do need to look back over the Unbreakable vision you have for yourself, and compare it to your current life.

- How do you spend your time?
- Who do you spend your time with?
- What interests do you pursue?
- Is your job sucking you dry and is there anything you can do about that?
- Is how you're living your life how you 'have' to live your life?
- Are there people in your life who reinforce an expression of who you might have once been but no longer are?
- What is the deepest desire that resides in your Unbreakable vision for yourself and is your life set up so that you can achieve it?

If there are mismatches between the two, you're going to have to reconcile that at some point — either by altering your Unbreakable vision or altering your life.

Your Unbreakable vision contains your values, either expressed overtly or subtly, and incongruence stifles those values. Sometimes the incongruence you find is there through no fault of your own — life happens and you've got to work with the hand you're dealt. Other times, the incongruence falls entirely on you due to your actions.

Thankfully, Unbreakable humans learn from every experience they have, and they put that experience to work for them so they can continue moving forward on their Unbreakable journey. The journey of becoming Unbreakable invites you to discover yourself and be fascinated, delighted, confused, and frustrated... and to learn from it all. It invites you to face yourself and all the BS you tell yourself that keeps you from becoming as powerful as you're capable of being. And it gives you ample practice in learning to give yourself grace, kindness, and love as you stumble and bumble your way through this one life you've got.

The decision to pack up and move to Utah allowed me to create a life I loved to live. I could not have become the person I am today without that one decision. To say it was the most impactful 'experiment' I've ever done in the name of becoming Unbreakable is an understatement. And it contained more fears, tears, frustrations, and enormous hurdles than I could ever have imagined.

And that's the thing: you *can't* know what is in store for you before you make the decisions you need to make. It's understandable that you want to know the risks and rewards ahead of time — especially when it comes to those big decisions in your life — and then make a sure-footed choice that is guaranteed to go well, or at least guaranteed to go pretty OK. But you just can't. And no one else can tell you what to do — it never ingrains quite as deep when someone tells you versus when you experience it yourself.

"One thorn of experience is worth a whole wilderness of warning" said James Russell Lowell, and like it or not, he's right.

Begin exploring your life and the choices you make each day. Explore your "I am" statements, which are the things you say that you are, and question all of them on occasion. "I am just not good at being disciplined to exercise." "I am always on the go, it's how I operate best." "I am old now, I can't do a marathon." Explore the little things and the big things. Explore your outlook on life. Explore why you do the things you do, and get to know this environment — inner and outer — that you're living in.

Tune in to the responses coming from your body, mind, spirit and anything else you believe is giving you guidance in your life. Sometimes, body responses that tell you if you're moving closer to alignment or incongruence feel so small and insignificant that you might at first carry on right past them — things like the inner glow of joy when you accomplish something challenging that you set your mind to do, or the slight sense of dread as you say 'yes' to something when you really would have liked to say 'no'.

Learn to slow down and lean into your curious compassion as you explore these responses. Spend time considering which external and internal signals could be contributing to this response occurring. Is it some unspoken 'you should do it this way' guideline for life that got imprinted on your brain long ago, or perhaps it's the way your social circle lives that is now rubbing off on how you live your life, even though the way they live isn't how you want to live. Now, it's the fun and terrifying part — do experiments with the intent to curate your life into greater alignment with your Unbreakable vision you have for yourself.

You can't possibly know if the outcome will be what you hoped, and while you can hedge your bets, consult with close people, read books to learn how to choose which actions to take, you're still going to have to take a leap of self-trust. However the experiment goes, learn from it and go on to the next experiment.

Keep track of your discoveries, insights, and experiment results in your Unbreakable Field Journal. You'll be glad to look back on them one day, not only to see how far you've come, but to note just how much wisdom you've accrued. If you need an extra pair of eyes to help you interpret the results you're finding, you can always reach out to me at my homes on the web, The Unbreakable Body (www.theunbreakablebody.com/) and Fit For Real Life (www.fitforreallife.com/).

There will come a point one day when it is actually 'too late'. And you have no idea when that will be. Please don't shackle yourself into your life or your body with 'too late's' that aren't real. Don't give up on your body and your experience of living in it because it seems too complicated or too difficult, and don't hand over your autonomy to anyone else. This is your life — embrace it, even that dang ankle tightness that has been bugging you for six months now. And decide you'll go on the journey of a lifetime, to become Unbreakable: an adventure that will take you more places than you could have dreamed and that will teach you more about yourself than you ever imagined.

Acknowledgments

You always hear authors mention how it takes a small army to bring a book to life. I didn't have an army, but I did have a tiny assembly of people who helped me get this book into your hands. Writing a book is one of the hardest projects I've ever taken on, and I wouldn't have made it to the finish line without the following people:

To my guy, Josh Madsen, who told me to "go write your book" a few years ago, and then helped to clear the way so I could. This would have remained a pipe dream were it not for you. Thank you for constantly reminding me that good things happen.

To my editor, Laura, I am so grateful for your masterful

editing skills, and your guidance in navigating the self-publishing world. Thank you for making me a better writer, and for getting me to stop taking so damn long to get to the meat of the story.

To my designer, Ronald, thank you for sharing your talents and expertise with me for this project. You were able to take my words and turn them into visuals that perfectly captured the essence of what I wanted to convey.

To my two early readers, Janine and Sarah, who took the time to read my writing and let me know if I had anything here worth pursuing further. Janine, your feedback in reading those early chapters was a gift and I am so grateful to you. Sarah, thank you as well for reading those early chapters and for always reminding me that this is just like quilt-making — take it one square a time.

Notes

1. Aldrich, M. (2016, January 22). Too much screen time is raising rate of childhood myopia [Blog post]. Retrieved from https://keck.usc.edu/too-much-screen-time-is-raising-rate-of-childhood-myopia/

2. Lerner, Li, Valdesolo, and Kassam (2014 September 22). Citation: Emotion and Decision Making. *Annual Review of Psychology*, 802. Retrieved from https://scholar.harvard.edu/sites/scholar.harvard.edu/files/jenniferlerner/files/emotion-and-decision-making.pdf?m=1450899163

3. Merriam-Webster. (n.d.) Problem. In *Merriam-Websiter.com dictionary*. Retrieved October 1 2020, from https://www.merriam-webster.com/dictionary/problem

4. Merriam-Webster. (n.d.) Opportunity. In *Merriam-Websiter.com dictionary*. Retrieved October 1 2020, from https://www.merriam-webster.com/dictionary/opportunity

5. Eagleman, D. (2017, October). Understanding the neuroscience that fuels creative thinking can make you more innovative. [Post]. LinkedIn. https://www.linkedin.com/pulse/understanding-neuroscience-fuels-creative-thinking-can-david-eagleman/

6. Dweck, C. (2007) *Mindset: The New Psychology of Success*. (Updated Edition) New York City, New York: Ballantine Books

7. Stanny. B (2014) *Sacred Success: A Course In Financial Miracles*. Dallas, Texas: BenBella Books

8. SEER Training Modules, Organization Of The Nervous System. U. S. National Institutes of Health, National Cancer Institute. 1 Oct 2021 Retrieved from https://www.training.seer.cancer.gov/anatomy/nervous/organization/

9. 1Fishman, Ballantyne, and Rathmell (2010) Bonica's Management of Pain. 3rd ed. Philadelphia, Pennsylvania: Lippincott Williams and Wilkins

10. Brinkjiki et al. (2014) Systematic literature review of imaging features of spinal degeneration in asymptomatic populations *AJNR. American journal of neuroradiology*, 36(4), 811-816. https://doi.org/10.3174/ajnr.A4173

11. Beattie, et al. (2005). Abnormalities identified in the knees of asymptomatic volunteers using peripheral magnetic resonance imaging. *Osteoarthritis and cartilage*, 13(3), 181-186. https://doi.org/10.1016/j.joca.2004.11.001

12. Connor et al. (2003). Magnetic resonance imagine of the asymptomatic shoulder of overhead athletes: a 5 year follow up study. *The American journal of sports medicine*, 31(5), 724-727. https://doi.org/10.1177/03635465030310051501

13. Bree, Dara. (2019 September 13) *A Causal Role for Long-Term Potentiation in Chronic Pain*. Retrieved from https://www.painresearchforum.org/news/124316-causal-role-long-term-potentiation-chronic-pain

14. Fehmi and Shor (2018 July19) *Open Focus*. Retrieved from https://openfocus.com/

15. He et al., (2015). Therapeutic play intervention on children's perioperative anxiety, negative emotional manifestation and postoperative pain: a randomized controlled trial. *Journal of advanced nursing*, 71(5), 1032-1043. https://doi.org/10.1111/jan.12608

16. Fehmi and Robbins (2010) *Dissolving Pain: Simple Brain-Training Exercises for Overcoming Chronic Pain.* Boulder, Colorado, USA: Trumpeter Books

17. Csikszentmihalyi, M. (2004, February). *Flow, the secret to happiness.* [Video]. TED Conferences. https://www.ted.com/talks/mihaly_csikszentmihalyi_flow_the_secret_to_happiness

18. Wolff J. (1986). *The law of bone Remodelling.* Berlin, Germany: Springer-Verlag

19. Myers, T. (2014). *Anatomy Trains: Myofascial Meridians for Manual and Movement Therapists 3rd Edition.* London, England: Churchill Livingstone

20. Dye, Scott F MD. (2005 July). The Pathophysiology of Patellofemoral Pain: A Tissue Homeostasis Perspective. *Clinical Orthopaedics and Related Research: July 2005 - Volume 436 - Issue - p 100-110* doi: 10.1097/01. blo.0000172303.74414.7d.

21. Dye, Scott F MD. (1996 April). The Knee as a Biologic Transmission With an Envelope of Function, *Clinical Orthopaedics and Related Research: April 1996 - Volume 325 - Issue - p 10-18.* Retrieved from https://journals.lww.com/clinorthop/Fulltext/1996/04000/The_Knee_as_a_Biologic_Transmission_With_an.3.aspx

22. Faulkner et al., (1993) Injury to skeletal muscle fibers during contractions: conditions of occurrence and prevention. *Physical therapy*, 73(12), 911-921. https://doi.org/10.1093/ptj/73.12.911

23. Mirkin G. & Hoffman M. (1978) *The Sports Medicine Book*. Boston, Massachusetts, USA: Little, Brown &Co

24. Mirkin, G. (2015 September 16). Why Ice Delays Recovery [Blog post]. Retrieved from https://www.drmirkin.com/fitness/why-ice-delays-recovery. html

25. Massery, M.,(2005). Musculoskeletal and neuromuscular interventions: a physical approach to cystic fibrosis. *Journal of the Royal Society of Medicine*. Supplement No 45, Volume 98, 55-62. Retrieved from http://www.masserypt.com/wp-content/uploads/2016/02/ Massery-RSM-article.vol-98-sup-45p.55-662005.pdf

26. Buckthorpe, M., Stride, M., & Della Villa, F., (2019 July 14). Assessing And Treating Gluteus Maximus Weakness - A Clinical Commentary. *International Journal of Sports Physical Therapy* 14(4): 655–669

27. Aagaard, P., & Andersen, J. L. (2010). Effects of strength training on endurance capacity in top-level endurance athletes. *Scandinavian journal*

of medicine & science in sports. 20 Suppl 2, 39-47. https://doi.org/10.1111/j.1600-0838.2010.01197.x

28. Ryan, C (2019). *Civilized To Death: The Price of Progress.* New York City, New York, USA: Avid Reader Press / Simon & Schuster

About the Author

Kate Galliett is the all-around powerhouse behind Fit For Real Life, where she's been writing about how to get fit for this one real life you've got since 2008. Helping people build their body to be strong, capable, and Unbreakable so they can live life as fully, deeply, and energetically as possible is the only thing Kate has ever cared about.

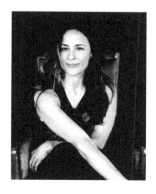

She's personally experienced what it's like to live life on the other side of the coin, where aches, pains, and a distrustful relationship with her body held her back from living life fully. And in fact, you wouldn't have recognized her then as compared to now. But over the span of 20 years, she's taken what she's learned on her own journey and taught it to others because the world is a better place if more people feel better.

Kate earned a B.S. in Exercise Science from Valparaiso University and went on to study a variety of certifications and trainings, all of which helped her curate the holistic approach she takes to body care today. In addition to her work with clients in-person and on her websites, she's coached at Nerd Fitness Adult Summer Camp, has been featured in Experience Life Magazine, Livestrong.com, and a variety of other publications. She lives in the great state of Utah where she can put her Unbreakable body to use for adventures in the mountains.

You can find Kate's work at www.fitforreallife.com and www.theunbreakablebody.com

Printed in Great Britain
by Amazon